Evaluating the Performance of the Hospital CEO

Third Edition

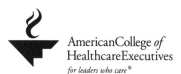

AmericanCollege *of*
HealthcareExecutives
for leaders who care ®

Health Administration Press

This publication is intended to provide accurate and authoritative information in regard to the subject matter covered. It is sold, or otherwise provided, with the understanding that the publisher is not engaged in rendering professional services. If professional advice or other expert assistance is required, the services of a competent professional should be sought.

The statements and opinions contained in this book are strictly those of the author(s) and do not represent the official positions of the American College of Healthcare Executives or of the Foundation of the American College of Healthcare Executives.

Copyright © 2004 by the Foundation of the American College of Healthcare Executives. Printed in the United States of America. All rights reserved. This book or parts thereof may not be reproduced in any form without written permission of the publisher.

08   07   06   05   04   5   4   3   2   1

Library of Congress Cataloging-in-Publication Data

American College of Healthcare Executives
    Evaluating the performance of the hospital CEO / 3rd ed.
        p. cm.
    Previous ed. published as: Evaluating the performance of the hospital CEO in a total quality management environment. Chicago, Ill.: American College of Healthcare Executives : American Hospital Association, c1993.
        Previous ed. cataloged under title.
        Includes bibliographical references.
        ISBN 1-56793-214-2 (alk. paper)
        1. Hospital administrators—Rating of.   2. Chief executive offers—Rating of. I. Evaluating the performance of the hospital CEO in a total quality management environment.   II. Title.
    RA971.E977 2003
    362.1'1'0684—dc22

                                                              2003060357

The paper used in this publication meets the minimum requirements of American National Standard for Information Sciences—Permanence of Paper for Printed Library Materials, ANSI Z39.48-1984. ∞ ™

Acquisitions manager: Audrey Kaufman; Project manager: Jane Williams; Cover design: Betsy Perez.

Health Administration Press
A division of the Foundation of the
    American College of Healthcare Executives
One North Franklin Street
Suite 1700
Chicago, IL 60606
(312) 424–2800

Contents

Introduction

> Evaluators draw their conclusions about performance from in-
> adequate data, informally gleaned impressions and pre-existing
> beliefs. Evaluatees often try to avoid blame rather than accept
> responsibility for those matters for which they are accountable.
> Many games are played with evaluation systems to ensure posi-
> tive conclusions.
>
> —*Cutt and Murray (2000)*

This monograph intends to help trustees and corporate officers charged with evaluating the performance of hospital chief executive officers (CEOs), and to help the CEOs themselves, avert the problems noted in the above quotation. In this monograph, we report the findings of a survey about current performance evaluation criteria conducted on a national sample of hospital CEOs affiliated with the American College of Healthcare Executives (ACHE). In addition, we relate 12 case studies derived from our interviews with hospital CEOs. The case studies reflect both the similarities and the differences in evaluation practices followed by not-for-profit, investor-owned, and government hospitals. These case studies were included in the monograph in hopes that readers may be able to take away lessons for and insights into enhancing their evaluation processes. Finally, we review the current literature that identifies benchmarks that evaluators can use in assessing their CEOs' performance. Ultimately, we hope that the information and views presented in this monograph will enhance the hospital CEO evaluation process and will pave the way for candid, useful appraisals.

CHAPTER OVERVIEW

Chapter 1 presents the general findings of the survey, while Chapter 2 focuses on CEOs of not-for-profit hospitals. Also in Chapter 2, more detailed information about the survey is conveyed and seven case studies based on interviews with hospital CEOs are provided. Chapter 3 considers investor-owned hospitals and presents two case studies—one featuring a CEO of a small rural hospital and another a CEO who manages a large urban hospital. Both of these CEOs report to a local board of trustees and a regional vice president of a large system. Chapter 4 details survey findings about three hospitals under government ownership, two of which are a small and a large district hospital and the other is a mid-sized hospital in the Veterans Administration system. The case studies discussed in the first four chapters include a copy of the actual forms used by the board (or supervisor) of those respective hospitals in evaluating their CEO's performance. We encourage you to consider them in either developing or modifying your own assessment form.

Chapter 5 summarizes some of the main processes followed by survey respondents. It also discusses the potential usefulness of benchmarking and 360-degree evaluations—tools that may become widely adopted in evaluating hospital CEOs more objectively and comprehensively. Chapter 6 presents the ACHE-suggested areas of CEO accountability by which a CEO's performance can be evaluated; the chapter includes questions for boards to consider in assessing each area. Appendix C (found at the end of this monograph) presents an annotated bibliography for additional information on the CEO evaluation topic.

THE HOSPITAL ENVIRONMENT

Healthcare futurists see many challenges for hospitals in the coming decade (Coile 2003), despite an upturn in inpatient admissions and occupancy rates at the time of this writing. Utilization, which was declining throughout the 1990s, is now increasing, and many hospitals are responding to this trend by reopening units or creating additional capacity by cutting length of stay. Staffing shortages, along with needed capital investment, pose major concerns for hospitals (Coile 2003). Hospitals are being challenged to transfer patients to other less-costly venues earlier, offer community outreach to the poor and underinsured, and improve the quality of the care they provide, all while being forced to battle for adequate reimbursement in a highly competitive marketplace.

The hospital remains the key health-restoring institution in the United States and in other countries. Physicians simply cannot provide proper medical care in isolation nor can aspiring healthcare practitioners obtain sufficient training apart from that available in hospitals. Research of all kinds is developed and tested in hospitals as well. The kingpin in the alliances formed between hospitals and laboratories, universities, government, and even entrepreneurial firms is the hospital. These alliances have meant new roles for hospitals. Communication and information-technology changes and new marketing efforts have stimulated the growth of interactive, long-distance patient care. Hospitals are expanding beyond their brick-and-mortar boundaries in an effort to completely enact their missions.

Also, hospitals are faced with the need to reconcile standard scientific healthcare practices with the innovations of the healing arts (such as alternative and complementary medicine) and the preferences of an increasingly sophisticated consumer population to whom information is now broadly available through the Internet. New types of facility and service lines have come into existence, posing new questions to hospitals about which opportunities to pursue and how to pursue them.

A renewed emphasis on safety and security is also affecting hospitals. As a result of quality-of-care research commissioned by the Institute of Medicine and various unfortunate medical incidents, patient-medication errors are now being studied. In the wake of terrorist attacks, hospitals are increasing their disaster relief and safety-preparedness activities. About four out of seven u.s. hospitals are now members of systems, in which evaluation by both superiors and peers is a standard part of the culture of control.

Finally, hospitals have grown in budgets and in numbers of patients treated, but not in number of beds. Likewise, hospitals' market orientation has increased the burden on managers, requiring greater efficiency from workers of all types. Sudden swings in patient censuses have exacerbated the already pressing shortage of nursing and other healthcare professionals. As a result, more and more hospitals are turning to private agencies to help them adequately staff their patient care units—a practice that contributes to increased costs.

To deal with these challenges, hospitals have had to become more entrepreneurial. However, ironically, hospitals today are less autonomous than ever: their medical practices, record-keeping systems, and business operations are increasingly subject to oversight from the government and other payers. These oversight agents want patient information to be standardized and transferable throughout systems so that outcomes and efficiencies can be compared and ultimately offered to the public. In turn, consumers can be given a chance to compare outcome information of one institution with that of another.

The leadership of a hospital has to transcend the role of mere "management" pursuing known goals with a mix of strategies and resources that is well understood and has been proven in practice. The hospital today must continually rethink and refine its goals, redevelop its strategies, battle for resources, and recreate itself organizationally. The hospital's best chance at survival is to have leaders who are as great as the challenges they face—that is, hospitals must be led by women and men of skill, knowledge, energy, integrity, creativity, and flexibility who are committed to their organization's mission and able to inspire the same commitment in others. Selecting such people for leadership positions and evaluating their performance is an indispensable task in today's hospital environment.

STUDY COMMITTEE

Peter Weil, Ph.D., FACHE, is the principal author of this third edition. Contributors to the survey include members of the 2001–2002 Research and Development Committee of ACHE. This committee includes the chair, George H. Perich, FACHE, of Fairmont General Hospital in Fairmont, West Virginia, and the following members:

- James A. Clindaniel, Jr., of O'Fallon Healthcare Center in O'Fallon, Illinois;
- Ralph Gabarro, CHE, of Mayo Regional Hospital in Dover-Foxcroft, Maine;
- Owen D. Garrick, M.D., of Novartis Pharmaceutical in San Ramon, California;
- Donald D. Hamilton, FACHE, of Cap Gemini Ernst & Young in Chicago;
- M. Ann Moser, FACHE, of Dennis R. Moser & Associates in Kingwood, Texas;

- Horace W. Murphy, FACHE, of Myersville, Maryland;
- the late Charles A. Rollberg, Ph.D., CHE;
- LCDR Mark J. Stevenson, FACHE, of TRICARE Lead Agent Central Region in Fort Carson, Colorado; and
- Steven C. Smith, FACHE, of the Mayo Clinic in Rochester, Minnesota.

In addition, the monograph was painstakingly reviewed by ACHE's executive leaders: Thomas C. Dolan, Ph.D., FACHE, CAE, president and chief executive officer, and Karen L. Hackett, FACHE, CAE, former executive vice president and chief operating officer.

Special acknowledgment must be given to the contributors of the 12 case studies in this edition. These CEOS spent approximately two hours each discussing the content and process of their evaluation. They were also generous in providing a copy of the template that their supervisors use to conduct their evaluation. Finally, we appreciate the survey responses, which we fielded in October 2001. The willingness of these executives to share their experience has contributed to our understanding of contemporary hospital CEO evaluation practices.

CHAPTER ONE

The Results of ACHE's National Survey of Hospital CEOs

To LEARN ABOUT the way hospital CEOs are being evaluated to-day, ACHE (through its Division of Research and Development) conducted a survey involving its CEO affiliates. In October 2001, a three-page fax survey was sent to 1,200 CEO affiliates. The survey requested information on the nature of these CEOs' performance evaluation, such as whether they are evaluated using preestablished written criteria and, if so, what specific criteria are used. In addition, the survey also asked if the CEOs' compensation is affected by the evaluation. Also included were several attitudinal questions concerning the perceived fairness of the evaluation and the appropriateness of the medical staff's and subordinates' involvement in the process (see Appendix A at the end of this monograph).

By the end of the study period—October 24, 2001—we received 363 responses for an overall response rate of 30 percent. A nonresponse analysis showed that respondents are not significantly different from nonrespondents in terms of hospital ownership (not for profit, investor owned, or government), size of hospital, or affiliation status with ACHE (Member, Diplomate, or Fellow). Also, no differences by gender were detected.

Table 1.1 shows that most hospitals evaluate their CEOs using pre-established written criteria. Fewer government hospitals—64 percent—have such criteria in place, and nearly all investor-owned hospitals—94 percent—have these criteria. (Even though no response bias by control was shown, the reader should be aware that the survey only yielded 34 respondents who manage investor-owned hospitals.) CEOS with written criteria in place are more likely to feel that their current appraisal process is fair (data not shown). Table 1.1 also shows that about 60 percent of the respondents permit such criteria to be modified during the evaluation period. In interviews we conducted, several CEOS stated that although the criteria can be changed, modification is a relatively rare phenomenon and is usually based on a larger environmental event such as the departure of a key group of physicians who admit many patients.

EVALUATION CRITERIA AND MEASURES

CEOS who are evaluated with preestablished written criteria were asked to indicate the criteria and specific measures used. The first set of criteria is *institutional success,* which reflects the CEO's accountabilities related to managing the hospital. Table 1.1 shows that under institutional success the most commonly used measure is fiscal management, which includes allocating financial, physical, and human resources. Using this measure, boards might consider whether healthcare services are produced in a cost-effective manner (that is, if efforts are made to employ economies while maintaining an acceptable level of quality) or whether an operating surplus is available. Over 90 percent of not-for-profit and government-owned hospitals evaluate their CEO using this measure, compared to 88 percent of investor-owned hospitals that use it.

Over 90 percent of CEOS in not-for-profit and investor-owned hospitals stated they are evaluated on customer satisfaction, compared to 74 percent of government-owned hospitals that use this measure. Using the customer satisfaction measure, evaluators might consider patient satisfaction scores in evaluating the CEO. Over 80 percent of hospitals use planning as a measure (e.g., updating the hospital's strategic plan), and about 80 percent of investor-owned and government hospitals use compliance with regulations (e.g., receiving JCAHO citations), with only 69 percent of not-for-profit hospitals citing it as a measure. Other measures used by at least 70 percent of hospitals are quality services (including consideration of the risk-adjusted mortality rate) and human resources management (including management of employee turnover, absenteeism, or results of employee attitude surveys).

In contrast to not-for-profit and investor-owned hospitals, government-owned hospitals more commonly evaluate their CEOS on leadership

TABLE 1.1: CEO PERFORMANCE EVALUATION CRITERIA
(IN PERCENTAGE)

	Not for Profit (n=252)	Investor Owned (n=34)	Government (n=83)	Chi Square p. sig.
Preestablished written criteria	76	94	64	**
	(n=192)	(n=32)	(n=54)	
Criteria can be modified during evaluation period	59	56	63	
Institutional Success				
Planning	83	81	83	
Human resources management	68	81	74	
Quality services	78	72	76	
Allocating financial/ physical/human resources	97	88	94	
Compliance with regulations	69	81	78	
Influencing legislation and regulations	35	25	31	
Promotion of the hospital	41	31	57	*
Customer satisfaction	91	97	74	***
Leadership	59	41	72	*
Community Health Status				
Processes to improve community health	28	9	24	
Outcomes to signify improvement	19	13	11	
Professional Role Fulfillment				
Continuing professional education	32	28	48	
Representing the profession	45	31	57	
Leadership/mentoring	19	16	33	*
Ethical methods to achieve goals	27	41	28	

*Chi square p. significant $p < .05$; **Chi square p. significant $p < .01$; ***Chi square p. significant $p < .001$

ability (e.g., conceptualizing a personal vision of healthcare delivery) and on promoting the hospital (e.g., having an effective communication and public relations program). The least commonly used measure, cited by a quarter to a third of respondents, is influencing legislation and regulations. Those that use this measure might consider how the CEO represents community health needs to legislators or how the CEO ensures that regulatory policies do not place unmanageable encumbrances on the hospital.

The second set of criteria is *community health status*. Here, only about a quarter of not-for-profit and government hospital CEOs told us they are evaluated on processes to improve community health, such as conducting health screening or immunization programs for the community. Even fewer—less than 20 percent—said their evaluations include consideration of community health status outcomes for infant mortality or teen pregnancy rates, for example.

The third and final set of criteria is *professional role fulfillment*. In contrast to the previous two sets, this focuses on the CEO's individual achievements. The most commonly used measure here is the CEO's role in representing the profession to civic and other organizations in the community. Over half of government hospitals (57 percent) and almost half of not-for-profit hospitals (45 percent) evaluate their CEOs on this criterion. With one exception, government hospitals more often use the measures under this criterion than do not-for-profit hospitals or investor-owned hospitals. Thus, 48 percent of government hospitals evaluate their CEO on his or her pursuit of continuing professional education, while 32 percent of not-for-profit hospitals use this measure and 28 percent of investor-owned hospitals use it.

Also, 33 percent of government hospitals, compared to less than 20 percent for the not for profits and investor owned, evaluate their CEOs on leadership including mentoring. In one measure under the professional role fulfillment criterion, ethical methods to achieve goals (e.g., complying with ACHE's Code of Ethics), more investor-owned hospitals evaluate their CEOs on this measure than do their not-for-profit and government counterparts: 41 percent for investor owned, compared to 27 percent for not for profits and 28 percent for government hospitals.

To get a better idea of how each set of criteria is appraised, respondents were asked to write in the specific measures that their boards (or supervisors) use. These written-in responses are summarized and presented in Table 1.2.

Planning	*(n=205)*
Goals/objectives/targets/strategic plan targets	134
Developing a plan	35
Operational measures (census, growth, discharges, budget)	20
Subjective	17
Other	6
Human Resources Management	*(n=165)*
Turnover	74
Employee satisfaction	60
Vacancy rate/deal with shortage/recruitment	17
Met goals	16
Subjective	12
Other	36
Quality	*(n=180)*
Quality indicators	50
Patient satisfaction	33
Plan objectives	27
JCAHO score	23
Benchmarks	13
Adverse incidents/lawsuits	11
Evidence-based medicine initiatives, practice guidelines	10
Other	51
Financial Management	*(n=228)*
Bottom line, profit margin, EBITDA, ROI	114
Meet budget/targets	102
Cash flow	14
Unit costs/productivity	14
Various indicators	12
Other	52
Compliance	*(n=165)*
JCAHO score	71
JCAHO accreditation	49
(Absence of) adverse citations/keep license	22
Compliance reporting/adherence to plan/goals/targets	21
Other external review	16
Other	15

(continued on following page)

The Results of ACHE's National Survey of Hospital CEOs

TABLE 1.2 *(continued)*

Advocacy	*(n=69)*
Advocacy efforts/involvement	21
Contacts with legislators	11
Subjective	11
Other	28
Promotion of the Hospital	*(n=97)*
Carrying out plan/goals/projects	27
Word of mouth/community support/image	14
Subjective	14
Other	45
Customer Satisfaction	*(n=201)*
Survey results	165
Goal/target/benchmark	35
Other	31
Leadership	*(n=117)*
Subjective	27
Targets, plan	22
Board/superior perception	18
Employee relationships/satisfaction/corporate culture	14
Other	54
Community Health Process	*(n=56)*
Program success/met targets	21
Participation in public health effort	10
Other	26
Community Health Outcomes	*(n=37)*
Planning objectives/targets/report	14
Clinical indicators	12
Other	16
Professional Education	*(n=73)*
Hours of CEU/programs attended	37
ACHE certification	13
Other	33
Representing the Profession	*(n=88)*
Activity in organizations	30
Community involvement/service	23
Number of appointments/positions	16
Other	20
Mentoring	*(n=41)*
Mentoring program/activity in firm	10
Annual target	7

TABLE 1.2 *(continued)*

Interns/residents	5
Management team redesign/team development	5
Other	17
Ethics	*(n=50)*
Corporate policy	13
Avoid unethical action/compliance problems/conflict	10
Compliance program/audit/review	10
Other	20

TABLE 1.3: CEO PERFORMANCE EVALUATION'S IMPACT ON
COMPENSATION (IN PERCENTAGE)

	Not for Profit (n=248)	Investor Owned (n=34)	Government (n=82)	Chi Square p. sig.
Salary	27	29	33	***
Bonus	18	9	26	
Both	50	50	24	
Neither	5	12	17	
TOTAL	100	100	100	

***Chi square p. significant p < .001

EVALUATION IMPACT ON COMPENSATION

CEOS who are evaluated based on preestablished written criteria were asked if the evaluation affected their compensation—that is, salary, incentive (bonus), or both. As Table 1.3 shows, significant differences are apparent between the three hospital-ownership types. The main difference is that nearly all types of not-for-profit hospital CEOS' compensation are somehow affected by the evaluation.

Conversely, a significantly higher proportion of the compensation of government hospital CEOS is not affected by the evaluation. For those affected, the effect on compensation, however, is confined to either salary or bonus, but not both.

TABLE 1.4: CEO PERFORMANCE EVALUATION WRITTEN-IN CRITERIA (IN NUMBER)*

No areas given, goals not cited	41
Areas given, goals cited	46
Annual goals/strategic plan objectives	31
Financial	22
Board/physician/employee relation and customer satisfaction	6
Compliance/quality/outcomes/patient satisfaction	6
Human resources	4
Community involvement	3
Mission	2
CEO behavior	1

*Reported by CEOS who are evaluated without preestablished criteria.

WRITTEN-IN EVALUATION CRITERIA

CEOS who are not evaluated on preestablished written criteria were asked to write in the criteria by which their performance is assessed. Table 1.4 shows that a large number of these CEOS (31) are evaluated on yearly goals set by the hospital. Another sizeable subset (22) stated they are evaluated on financial outcomes. Forty-one respondents did not indicate any criteria or candidly wrote in that their evaluation is "subjective."

ATTITUDES OF CEOS

Lastly, the survey posed four attitudinal probes to gauge CEOS' opinions about their evaluation. CEOS were asked to answer by indicating whether they agree, disagree, or are neutral about a statement (see Table 1.5). The first question is "My current appraisal is fair." Over 80 percent of those in not-for-profit and investor-owned hospitals stated that they feel their evaluation is, indeed, fair. However, a significantly lower percentage—71 percent—of CEOS in government hospitals agreed.

The second statement is "CEOS should be evaluated by others on the management team." Table 1.5 data show that over half of CEOS in all types

	Not for Profit (n=249)	Investor Owned (n=34)	Government (n=82)	Chi Square p. sig.
My current appraisal is fair:				*
Disagree	4	3	11	
Neutral	12	9	18	
Agree	84	88	71	
CEOS should be evaluated by others on the management team:				
Disagree	25	26	29	
Neutral	24	18	18	
Agree	51	56	52	
CEOS should be evaluated by physicians on the hospital medical staff:				
Disagree	31	41	29	
Neutral	22	15	23	
Agree	47	44	48	
No one can really appreciate what I accomplished for the hospital:				
Disagree	75	71	68	
Neutral	12	23	13	
Agree	13	6	19	

*Chi square p. significant $p < .05$

of hospitals feel that they should be evaluated by others on their management team. CEOS have considerable interest in obtaining feedback from their subordinates. Related to this second probe is the third one: "CEOS should be evaluated by physicians on the hospital medical staff." A slightly reduced percentage—less than 50 percent—of respondents agree with this idea. However, a sizeable minority—between 29 and 41 percent—disagree with physicians' involvement in the CEO's evaluation.

The fourth statement is "No one can really appreciate what I accomplished for the hospital." We learned that the vast majority—between two thirds and three quarters—of respondents feel that others can appreciate their accomplishments for the hospital, and most of the remaining respondents chose to be neutral.

CONCLUSION

This chapter outlines the results of a performance evaluation survey on ACHE-affiliated CEOS. The preestablished, written evaluation criteria reported by the CEOS mostly focus on the accountabilities of the CEO to the hospital and less on the CEOS' roles in improving community health. Fulfilling professional roles and pursuing continuing education fell somewhere between the institutional success and community health status criteria. The CEOS' performance evaluation does affect their compensation, and those who are not evaluated on specific written criteria state that their evaluations depend on achieving goals set by the hospital. By and large, CEOS perceive their evaluations to be fair, but fewer CEOS in government-owned hospitals agree with this statement.

CHAPTER TWO

Evaluating the CEO of the Not-for-Profit Hospital

I N THIS CHAPTER, we examine the CEO evaluation process in not-for-profit hospitals. The CEOs' survey responses were divided into three categories by hospital size. Classifying responses allows us to determine if the findings discussed in Chapter 1 are a result of size rather than control. Small hospitals are defined as those with less than 100 beds, medium-size hospitals are those with 100 to 199 beds, and large hospitals are those that have 200 beds or more.

Table 2.1 shows that preestablished written criteria for the ceo's evaluation are in place in about three-quarters of all not-for-profit hospitals, regardless of the hospital's size. In addition, these criteria are modifiable during the evaluation period in over half of the hospitals. The evaluation criteria are more or less similar among small, medium, and large hospitals. CEOs of small hospitals are evaluated based on their compliance with regulations (80 percent) and their continuing professional education (43 percent) more so than are their counterparts in medium and large organizations. On the other hand, CEOs of medium-sized hospitals are evaluated more on their leadership activities, such as mentoring, compared to ceos of small and large hospitals.

Table 2.2 indicates that nearly all not-for-profit hospital ceos get compensated based on their evaluation; for about half of all not-for-profit CEOs, the evaluations are tied to both salary and bonus. However, a higher percentage of small hospitals (39 percent) exclusively tie their ceos' evaluation to salary, compared to that done by medium and large hospitals (18 and 22 percent, respectively).

TABLE 2.1: NOT-FOR-PROFIT HOSPITAL CEO PERFORMANCE EVALUATION CRITERIA, BY ORGANIZATIONAL SIZE (IN PERCENTAGE)

	Less than 100 Beds (n=97)	Between 100 and 199 Beds (n=69)	200 Beds and More (n=86)	Chi Square p. sig.
Preestablished written criteria	77	78	74	
	(n=75)	(n=54)	(n=63)	
Criteria can be modified during evaluation period	65	55	55	
Institutional Success				
Planning	83	89	78	
Human resources management	73	59	70	
Quality services	71	78	87	
Allocating financial/physical/ human resources	95	98	98	
Compliance with regulations	80	61	63	*
Influencing legislation and regulations	37	37	30	
Promotion of the hospital	49	37	33	
Customer satisfaction	91	85	95	
Leadership	64	52	60	
Community Health Status				
Processes to improve community health	35	20	27	
Outcomes to signify improvement	19	19	21	
Professional Role Fulfillment				
Continuing professional education	43	37	14	***
Representing the profession	51	46	38	
Leadership/mentoring	12	31	16	*
Ethical methods to achieve goals	28	26	27	

*Chi square p. significant p < .05; ***Chi square p. significant p < .001

	Less than 100 Beds (n=96)	Between 100 and 199 Beds (n=67)	200 Beds and More (n=85)	Chi Square p. sig.
Salary	39	18	22	n.s.*
Bonus	13	21	22	
Both	46	54	51	
Neither	3	7	5	
TOTAL	100	100	100	

* not significant p > .05

Table 2.3 illustrates that not-for-profit CEOs' opinions about their evaluations are similar, regardless of the size of their hospitals. Over 80 percent agree to the attitudinal probe "My current appraisal is fair." Moreover, about half of the CEOs also agree to the statement "CEOs should be evaluated by others on the management team." (The smaller percentage of medium-size hospital CEOs who agree to this probe can be considered an anomaly.) To the statement "CEOs should be evaluated by physicians on the hospital medical staff," the agreement ranges between 41 and 55 percent; the disagreement to the statement is similar across the board at 29, 34, and 31 percent. The final attitudinal probe is "No one can really appreciate what I accomplished for the hospital," which yielded a high proportion of disagreement. Apparently, these not-for-profit hospital CEOs believe that people do appreciate their contribution to their respective organizations.

CASE STUDIES

The seven case studies presented below reflect the diversity of CEO-evaluation processes among not-for-profit hospitals. The seven hospitals featured in this section vary in bed size, ranging from a 25-bed hospital in northwestern Montana to a 407-bed hospital in northeastern Texas.

Table 2.3: Not-for-Profit Hospital CEOs' Perceived Attitude About Performance Evaluation (in percentage)

	Less than 100 Beds (n=96)	Between 100 and 199 Beds (n=67)	200 Beds and More (n=86)	Chi Square p. sig.
My current appraisal is fair:				
Disagree	5	6	1	
Neutral	14	10	12	
Agree	81	84	87	
CEOs should be evaluated by others on the management team:				
Disagree	26	22	26	**
Neutral	18	40	17	
Agree	56	38	56	
CEOs should be evaluated by physicians on the hospital medical staff:				
Disagree	29	34	31	
Neutral	16	24	28	
Agree	55	43	41	
No one can really appreciate what I accomplished for the hospital:				
Disagree	68	75	82	
Neutral	14	11	10	
Agree	17	14	8	

**Chi square p. significant p < .01

Included in each case study is a profile that states the size of the hospital's community, the major industries in the area, and the hospital's sources of revenue. In addition, the case studies address the structure of each hospital's CEO performance evaluation—that is, what methods are used, how the evaluation is related to the compensation package, and how the CEO expects his or her evaluation to change in the future. The case studies also offer advice from CEO interviewees on improving the CEO evaluation process. Note that details in the case studies were accurate as of the writing of this monograph; they may have changed in the interim.

Case Study 2.1

Organization: St. John's Lutheran Hospital, Libby, Montana
CEO: Richard L. Palagi, CHE
Size: 25 beds
Community Profile: St. John's Lutheran is a 25-bed critical access hospital that is located within a service area of 18,000 people; its primary service area consists of 14,000 people. The main industries in the area are lumber and mining, but a recreation sector that includes river guiding and floating and fly fishing is growing. In this county, which is considered the second poorest in the entire state of Montana, healthcare is the largest, consistent, private employer. The community is fairly remote: the nearest large hospital is located 90 miles away (in Kalispell) and the nearest major medical center is located 160 miles away (in Spokane).
Sources of Revenue: 55 percent Medicare, 15 percent Medicaid, 15 percent commercial insurance, 15 percent self-pay. The number of uninsured but working patients is growing.

Rick Palagi, CEO of St. John's, has been with the hospital for eight years. For the first five years, he served as CEO under a contract-management agreement that the hospital had with Brim Associates, a consulting firm that provides hospitals with contract executives. Three years ago, the board asked him to develop a job description for himself and an evaluation tool that the board could use. He did exactly that, and St. John's board has been using this evaluation tool since its development.

At St. John's, the CEO is evaluated using eight criteria (see Appendix B at the end of this monograph for a copy of this evaluation form). One area of performance that is not currently evaluated under this tool is the CEO's involvement in legislation and regulations. Because Rick currently sits on the Montana Hospital Association's board and is a spokesperson for federal contacts, he thinks this area should be added to his evaluation.

A 360-degree evaluation is part of the CEO appraisal at St. John's. The 360 involves feedback from the board; the senior vice presidents who report directly to the CEO; other direct reports, including the CEO's administrative assistant; and the heads of rehabilitation, radiology, primary care, and urgent care. In addition, questionnaires about the CEO's performance are distributed to the medical staff and all department managers. In the future, Rick would like to include community leaders in evaluating his performance. Leaders may include the heads of the local chamber of commerce, the community college, the Economic Development Council, leading businesspeople in the area, and the county commissioners who oversee public health. Currently, Rick and the board are not ready to pursue this avenue.

In addition to being evaluated based on criteria on the performance evaluation form, the CEO is also evaluated based on achievement of specific goals listed on the hospital's annual strategic plan. Accompanying these goals are several dashboard indicators, including financial, quality, and satisfaction measures, that identify the CEO's leadership abilities. The patient satisfaction measure is an aggregate of scores for all acute care provided within the year as well as ancillary, laboratory, radiology, rehabilitation, home health, and physicians' satisfaction with senior managers and the hospital itself. Combining the results of these measures, the board, in a subjective way, then determines the CEO's performance accordingly: needs improvement, satisfactory—meets targets, and satisfactory—exceeds targets.

Rick's compensation is not determined by a fixed schedule. Instead, the board uses as a guide the Montana Hospital Association's published statistics on salaries and bonuses for leaders of hospitals of similar size and the hospital's ability to fund. The board also relies on its subjective sense of the appropriate amount by which to set Rick's salary and bonus for the coming year. The entire 12-member board is involved in his evaluation. As mentioned, Rick wants to include a community component to his evaluation, but he also wants to continue to use the form to see changes from year to year.

St. John's board conducts a self-evaluation that mirrors many of the measures used for appraising its CEO. Rick notes that the current self-evaluation form is the second version; the first form did not meet the board's needs. In general, Rick believes that his current chair—a former registered technician and nurse but now a successful businesswoman—really understands healthcare and its complexities. The chair is elected to serve for one year, a term that Rick would like to see extended to two years in the future. Because of a current community-level health issue (18 percent of the area's population has been diagnosed as suffering from asbestosis), Rick expects the current chair to remain in office for four years.

Rick's advice to boards for improving their CEO evaluations is as follows:

I think you would want to look at evaluation as a system, a set of processes and measures that would key from the mission, vision, and strategic plan. Ideally, you would try to be consistent in the principles you applied. Some of the individual items would be tracked at all levels consistently, including the department level, the enterprise level, and the governance level. If my measurements are consistent with what department managers are getting measured on, then I believe we have a much better chance of being cohesive and in pursuit of similar outcomes. It's easier said than done. We conduct 360-degree evaluations on all of our managers; we use a similar collection tool in terms of the 1-to-5 kinds of scores.

Case Study 2.2

Organization: Atlantic General Hospital, Berlin, Maryland
President/CEO: Barry G. Beeman
Size: 62 beds
Community Profile: Atlantic General Hospital is a 62-bed, freestanding facility (the only one within a 30-mile radius) that serves the second largest city in Maryland—Ocean City, with a population that swells in the summer to 400,000. The emergency room cares for 22,000 patients per year. The hospital serves Worcester county, which has a population of 70,000; its primary service area has 42,000 people. Overall, about 40 percent of the population are over 65 years old. Worcester is the fastest growing county in Maryland—its population increases by 20 percent each year. Its main industries are tourism and poultry farming, but the hospital is the county's second largest employer, employing 450 people. Economically, the community is doing well. The hospital has a separate foundation with its own board, which is composed of influential people in the community who are dedicated to raising funds to help the hospital meet its goals. Fundraising activities of the board include conducting capital campaigns, coordinating planned givings, and hosting annual fundraisings.
Sources of Revenue: 52 percent Medicare, 1 percent Medicaid, 28 percent commercial insurance, 17 percent HMO, 2 percent self-pay

Only eight years old, Atlantic General Hospital started with a CEO who was under a management contract. After that contract, the hospital hired its current CEO, Barry Beeman, who has been in the position for three years. With the board's executive committee, Barry establishes his annual performance evaluation criteria, which include various measures such as strategic planning, finance, community relations, and employee relations. Together, Barry and the board review the objectives and then prioritize them. The whole board then approves the objectives. The objectives can be modified based on circumstances that arise over the course of the year. The challenge that currently confronts Atlantic General's leadership is in trying to figure out the best way to operationalize the specific measures—that is, how to determine if an objective is met and how to rank order each objective. Barry feels (and he thinks his board chair agrees) that some objectives are more important than others and that the ability to achieve each objective needs to be rated. One criterion for evaluation is a general administration accountability, which includes leadership areas such as communication.

At the time of our interview, Barry admitted that the verdict was still out on whether the criteria were fair; this is because the evaluation tool was only two months old then. Because of the history of the board chair and the former CEO, a number of role issues have been brought out, issues that are being resolved during Barry's tenure. Clearly, the evaluation tool is derived from the CEO's job description, but the CEO's objectives do not parallel those criteria that the board considers in its evaluation. Some accountabilities are similar, but there is minimal overlap.

Because the 19 board members include 4 staff physicians, Barry feels that the medical staff's personal views of him are voiced in the evaluation. He is supportive of a 360-degree evaluation, but at the time of our interview none of his direct reports were being given a chance to evaluate his performance. In the future, Barry's subordinates will likely evaluate him as will those on the foundation board (influential members of the community) and even the hospital's community partners. Barry's evaluation affects the percentage increase in his base pay and bonus. He has a five-year contract.

In the future, Barry expects that his evaluation will change in the following ways:

> I think we'll definitely put some value on each accountability. We'll tie the evaluation results into the actual percentage given for the base salary

increase and for the bonus increase. We will definitely look at expanding the constituencies that have input into this process, and we'll get more formalized as we move forward. I think I have a very good sense of where accountabilities will move in the next year or two. As you know, the way healthcare is changing, I don't think anybody will know what accountabilities will be needed five years from now. For example, bioterrorism over the course of a year might become front and center. But I don't know if that will ever become an accountability in itself; it might fall under administrative leadership—the ability to react to necessary issues in a responsible way.

Barry's advice to boards who are deciding on improving their CEO's evaluation is threefold:

1. Communication is key. Each side needs to listen to avoid coming into negotiations with set expectations.
2. Accountabilities have to be realistic. A 10 percent operating surplus today isn't going to happen.
3. The objectives should not be etched in stone. Healthcare is too volatile an environment for that.

Case Study 2.3

Organization: Bay Area Medical Center, Marinette, Wisconsin
President/CEO: David A. Olson, FACHE
Size: 115 beds
Community Profile: The hospital has 115 licensed beds. Its primary service area has 35,000 people, and its secondary service area has 70,000. The hospital's net revenue is $75 million per year. The community of Marinette is a blue-collar town. Its major industries are paper manufacturing, ship building, and farming.
Sources of Revenue: 40 percent Medicare, 10 percent Medicaid, 50 percent commercial insurance

Dave Olson, FACHE, was selected interim CEO of Bay Area Medical Center in the spring of 1999; by the fall of the same year, he was appointed as the permanent CEO. At that time, the board gave the CEO a bonus in a post-hoc way. But Dave was interested in a compensation system that was structured. He believes that incentives should be set forth at the beginning of the year as it allows emotions to be removed from compensation decisions. Therefore, in 2000, Dave initiated a system that would bring more rigor. He adapted the form published by the Iowa Hospital Association entitled "The CEO Annual Evaluation Guide," which uses a grid to assess six major areas. Admittedly, the grid Dave developed is a subjective assessment tool, but at least it provides a basis for discussion.

Both Dave and the board's CEO Performance and Compensation Subcommittee complete the grid. The subcommittee consists of four board members; prior to the CEO's review, the subcommittee discusses their findings with the full nine-member board. In times of stressful situations, the grid helps the board remember that they assessed the CEO as doing a good job. Moreover, the grid offers an opportunity to talk about new activities that can be initiated and provides a chance to discuss matters that are not going well. The evaluation criteria are changeable over the course of a year, depending on environmental changes. For example, if a large influx of physicians were to join the staff, some adjustments may have to be made in some of the targets previously established.

Apart from the grid, which determines his base salary level, Dave developed a list of major goals that forms the basis of his incentive. For example, in 2001, Dave had five goals in the areas of quality, customer service, operational efficiency, financial goals, and progress toward achieving the strategic plan. Each of these goals is evaluated at three levels: (1) minimum threshold, (2) target, and (3) outstanding. For example, in the quality goal, Dave used an issue of concern to the hospital—medication-administration accuracy. In addition to Dave's goals, the board includes six goals that can be more subjectively measured. Two goals are improving the satisfaction of middle managers and getting the new building opened by a certain month. These goals are not changeable during the course of a year. Finally, Dave adds two personal goals to the list that tell the board the other objectives he is pursuing. For example, he is interested in developing a corporate culture, a goal that has continuing-education implications; this may later translate to a hospital goal. Another goal is his plan to pursue a doctorate degree.

The entire hospital staff uses a 360-degree evaluation system, except for the CEO, but this may change in the future. Changing it would entail the CEO asking the CFO and the COO to evaluate his performance.

The board has a pay philosophy: senior executives should be salaried at the 65th percentile of salaries paid to executives of similar-sized hospitals in the region. To this end, the board commissions Health Care

Compensation Strategies, a firm based in Minneapolis, Minnesota, that conducts a survey to assess CEO tenure, the market, and the salary range within the market. For new CEOs, the board pays between 80 and 90 percent of the median salary; for more tenured CEOs, the target is to pay from 91 to 110 percent of the median. This is the decision into which subjectivity enters. At Bay Area Medical Center, the bonus opportunity is 8 percent for minimum threshold achievement, 16 percent for target achievement, and 24 percent for outstanding achievement.

In general, not many clinical indicators are currently being used in Dave's evaluation; the future may be different however. The current board seems comfortable with financial indicators and not with clinical indicators, given that they are mostly businesspeople. Dave would likely use internal hospital issues to guide the selection of clinical indicators. One current hospital internal issue can serve as a clinical indicator: the hospital's rate of readmissions for chronic congestive heart failure patients compared with readmission benchmarks published by the Michigan Hospital Association. In addition, at present, community health is not considered in Dave's evaluation.

The board's self-evaluation is not as structured as the CEO's. In the future, the board may use the CEO's performance evaluation criteria as a guide for board development. Thus, future clinical and quality goals set for the CEO may become educational opportunities for the mostly financially driven board. Also, Dave would like to see measures of community health incorporated into his evaluation in the future. Here is Dave's take on how his evaluation will change and who will effect these changes:

I think that if this is going to change, it will probably be [because of] things that I'm going to have to bring forward. The steps I see are really a way to use the CEO's performance evaluation as a way to do board development. If our board's primary interest in the past has been the financial performance of the organization, then I feel that by introducing concepts of clinical performance, quality performance as part of my own goals will help them broaden their understanding that their role as a board is beyond that of fiduciary. Part of this is taking small steps. I foresee in this next year doing more in clinical outcomes and introducing some of the things that are going to improve the health of our community beyond acute care. People come here and get well after they leave. We have a high incidence of cardiac problems; we're up here in the cheese belt, and diets aren't the best. I think our board will view that as 'well, that's great as long as you're meeting your financial goals but....' I think introducing that as a goal is going to be a step forward.

The following is Dave's advice to boards on improving their CEO evaluation and other messages:

First, I'd say to have at least some element of structure to it. The reason is that it creates a situation where there aren't any surprises—surprises for the board or surprises for the CEO. I think that you hear these horror stories about CEOs who think they're doing a good job and then all of a sudden something happens, and the board sits them down and they're told they're not doing a good job. But then from the board's side—and I think this is one of the things that our board has always wanted to make sure of—they don't want to find out that they're behind in compensation. I think boards hate it when they lose a CEO. In fact, things have been going very well up here for our hospital and for me. You know I got the Young Administrator of the Year Award in March, and now I think our board is just very concerned, 'Boy, are you going to leave?' And my sense is 'you all are paying me fairly.' That's something they need to work toward. I don't think they should reward me anything extra because of that, as long as compensation is fair. Even if I would go and take another job someday, they're going to have their salary range at the market and they'll be able to find someone else. That way, the board doesn't have a surprise

The other thing I feel strongly about is [that] you have this one time a year when you collect all the data and you talk about your performance at each board meeting. I try to have our hospital board see the performance of our senior management team so they understand what all of us are doing to meet our goals. And that's where I feel like a solid strategic plan has been absolutely critical because all of the goals I have for myself and for my senior managers get pulled from the strategic plan. That's what we ought to be spending our time working on. And if we're working on something else, it ought to be in the strategic plan; if it's not, then we ought not to be working on it.

Case Study 2.4

Organization: Keokuk Health Systems, Keokuk, Iowa
CEO: Allan W. Zastrow, FACHE
Size: 120 beds

Community Profile: Keokuk Health Systems has a hospital with 120 beds, 20 skilled-care beds, and a 14-bed psychiatric unit. In addition to the hospital, the system has a physician clinic, a durable medical equipment subsidiary, an insurance company, and a foundation. The budget for the entire system is approximately $50 million. Keokuk is tucked in the southeast corner of Iowa on the Mississippi river with a population of about 13,000. The hospital serves a population of about 30,000, and 20 percent of its patients come from Illinois and as many come from Missouri. The community has a diverse industrial base; it has corn mills, a large rubber plant for automobile parts, several foundries, and a train car manufacturer.

Sources of Revenue: 55 percent Medicare, 13 percent Medicaid, 27 percent commercial insurance, 5 percent self-pay

Allan Zastrow, FACHE, has been with Keokuk for 14 years. He is evaluated annually by five members of the system's boards' CEO Evaluation Committee. There are five boards in the entire system, and each member of the five boards is given the CEO appraisal form to complete. The CEO Evaluation Committee compiles the results and discusses them with the CEO. This form was developed recently by the system board, and it includes criteria that the board members believe are most important in the CEO's evaluation. Allan developed the previous form. In the past, Allan was evaluated on professional development, but this criterion has dropped out, as Allan says, "probably because the board saw that I was pursuing this steadily." Allan adds, "[I'm] not uncomfortable with the current form. Really, it serves as a basis for a good discussion and developing an open relationship between my board and me." At the time of the interview, community health improvement, although part of the system's mission, was not reflected in the CEO evaluation; Allan thinks it should be, however.

Keokuk does not employ a 360-degree assessment for the CEO. Because the board has ultimate responsibility for the organization, Allan thinks lacking the 360 is okay. In the past, medical staff were offered the opportunity to comment on the CEO's performance, but few did. Today, the medical staff's views are expressed through physician board members. Allan believes that the employees' voice is heard through surveys conducted routinely.

The evaluation affects Allan's salary: his increase depends on the evaluation he receives. There is no limit to the increase, and each year the board sets a target range—in 2000, it was 3 percent and in 2001, it was 6 percent. Allan's incentive compensation is tied to achieving hospital objectives, which are absolute targets set at the beginning of the year. He appreciates the constructive feedback he gets from his evaluation. Although the board gets a quarterly progress report on the hospital's objectives in his evaluation, Allan only has one conversation about them each year. This is alright with him because he gets informal feedback at the many meetings he attends with board members. He does not feel he needs to go over these objectives more often.

As for the future, Allan expects that finances will be more heavily emphasized then because of reduced Medicare payments. Also, he expects that after some board education on the issue, the board will establish community health objectives for him in this area. Allan offers the following advice to boards:

> Right now, CEO evaluation is often looked on as a necessary evil. But it should be looked on as a process improvement opportunity—a way to establish relationships and talk about what's important. [Boards should] identify in their own minds what it is they think is important for their CEO to be doing and their organizations to be doing and base [the evaluation] on that. I think to take a form and go through and fill something out probably doesn't meet much of a need if it's not relevant to what that particular organization and that particular board wants. Just having been in the field for quite a while, I see that disconnect as one that's fairly hazardous for CEOs. If you're measured on things that first off you didn't know about or are not really relevant to what you're doing, there's a fairness issue there.... Too often, and I don't blame boards, they think it's a necessary evil—'let's get it done, tell him you're doing OK or we want him to do this or that. I think it's really a process, a part of the performance improvement environment of every organization. CEO evaluation is probably one of the more important pieces [on which] to establish a relationship and talk about what is there. It doesn't really matter what the forms say; you're going to get the input on the form as a form. But really, the performance improvement type of mentality of where you're going as an organization and what you want the CEO to contribute to that is probably the most important part.

Allan agrees that the evaluation form is a sensible springboard in making sure that CEOs and their boards are seeing eye to eye and that board members are being candid with the CEO:

Many board members are not trained to do performance appraisals. A lot of these people are lay people who may not have done them in their own organization. And even if they have, they do them differently, and you have the different forces of the medical staff and the community and those types of things. So I think they come at it from a very uninformed or very different background than the healthcare arena. I think that is a real big potential for problems. Complexity makes it especially difficult in the performance appraisal of the hospital CEO.

Case Study 2.5

Organization: Wadley Regional Medical Center, Texarkana, Texas
President/CEO: James A. Summersett, III, FACHE
Size: 407 beds
Community Profile: Wadley Regional Medical Center is a Level-II trauma center that has 407 beds and currently staffs for 250 patients. Its annual revenues are in excess of $180 million. Located in Texarkana, Texas, with a population of 75,000, Wadley has a primary service area of 137,195 people; its secondary service area has 125,280. Texarkana sits in the midpoint of a triangle formed by Little Rock, Arkansas; Shreveport, Louisiana; and Dallas, Texas. Healthcare is its number one industry, but other employers are in the area, including the U.S. Army (which has a depot in the community where components of cruise missiles are manufactured), International Paper, Georgia Pacific, and Cooper Tire and Rubber Company.
Sources of Revenue: 48 percent Medicare, 12 percent Medicaid, 10 percent commercial, 22.7 percent HMO and PPO, 7.3 percent self-pay

Jim Summersett, FACHE, has been CEO at Wadley for a little over three years. (He has a three-year rolling contract.) He has used the same evaluation instrument for 12 years. To Jim, it seems that each hospital he works for does not have its own CEO evaluation form, so they appreciate the fact that Jim has developed his own. For his part, Jim tracks his performance on each of the 82 items (see Appendix B). Once a year, the entire board completes the executive evaluation tool anonymously; then, the results are tallied by the board chair. The results are used by the Compensation Committee (i.e., the three officers of the board) and influence the amount of the CEO's salary increase. Until a couple of years ago, the opportunity for increase was 0 to 8 percent; now, no limits are specified. Jim's bonus is determined by another set of criteria—that is, achieving the hospital's corporate objectives.

Jim thinks that the criteria are appropriate but that some board members feel unable to answer all the items such as "Budgets personal time well"; in that case, they leave the item blank. The items are all subjective. The board can add an item or two to the criteria, but for the most part the 82 items have remained the same. The board also conducts its own self–evaluation, but any criteria on their own evaluation that resemble those in the CEO's evaluation are purely coincidental.

Given that the whole organization is moving toward 360-degree evaluations, Jim expects that his evaluation in the future will be a 360-degree one, with his six direct reports providing feedback. This might have already been implemented had the board not stumbled on whom to consider as Jim's peers each time the matter was discussed. The criteria might change, but if they do, Jim would like to continue using the current form for continuity's sake. Several years ago, he began to give a brief, four- to five-item feedback to his direct reports quarterly. He got the idea from his children's report cards. That evaluation worked well, and Jim might reinstitute it. In the future, he would like more formal feedback:

> There's a lot of water that goes under the bridge in a year. If you're not getting feedback over a 12-month period, you can get way off base with one of these issues until you sit down with the tool. I think that's a general criticism of the whole process. An annual evaluation is probably not adequate. We would never think about putting our kids in school and giving them a grade at the end of a year.... We don't put a patient in and decree their condition at the end of a hospital stay.

Jim's advice to boards is as follows:

> Communicate openly and often. And recognize that nobody on the board has the scope of responsibility anywhere near of what I do or the complexity that healthcare brings in general.

Case Study 2.6

Organization: Central DuPage Health System, Winfield, Illinois
President/CEO: Donald C. Sibery, FACHE
(*Author's note:* On November 27, 2002, Mr. Sibery resigned from his position.)

Size: 385 beds

Community Profile: Central DuPage is a vertically integrated system with a flagship hospital of 385 beds, a physician organization of 85 primary care and convenient care providers, 5 convenient care sites, a lifecare facility with 250 independent living units, 75 assisted living units, 210-bed skilled nursing facility, and a home health agency. The hospital has 750 physicians on staff and 4,300 full-time and part-time employees. It provides primary, secondary, and tertiary care to the 1 million or so residents of DuPage County, Illinois. The primary service area has 197,274 people, and the secondary service area has 446,520 people. The community is affluent and hosts a number of high-tech industries, including Lucent, Tellabs, and Motorola. The hospital has joint ventures with a nearby hospital and health system.

Sources of Revenue: 36 percent Medicare, 5 percent Medicaid, 3 percent commercial insurance and Blue Cross, 51 percent HMO, 5 percent self-pay

Don Sibery, FACHE, developed the criteria that at the time of this interview were used in his performance evaluation. He used the position description that had been developed for the board by Heidrick and Struggles, an international consultancy, in their search for a CEO, and he augmented the form by borrowing from other organizations and executives. Don's view is that the present evaluation form covers between 90 and 95 percent of the CEO's core competencies.

The evaluation form actually has three versions: (1) one for board members, (2) the other for medical staff leaders, and (3) another for senior executive staff. The CEO's review is conducted by the Executive Committee of the board. The chair of the board summarizes all the surveys and then gives this summary to the Executive Committee. The full board discusses the CEO's performance. Evaluation of the CEO involves not only the process described above but also includes two other elements: appraisal of the achievement of corporate objectives and two memos from the CEO describing achievement of personal objectives for the prior year and proposed personal objectives for the coming year. Personal objectives might include items such as incorporating more spontaneous leadership (e.g., drop-in conversations) into management relationships, developing relationships with other health systems, developing benchmarks to aid in accountability measurement, incorporating performance improvement in work life, and improving personal fitness. Don notes that when he began his tenure six years ago, his goals were much more ambitious and unrealistic. Over the years, the Executive Committee has asked him to rank order his objectives; sometimes, they have even asked him to delete some.

In sum, Don's annual personal objectives involve a process of negotiation with the board. In contrast, the CEO evaluation form remains the same from year to year. In addition, Don works with a coach:

> I happen to be a personal fan and user of coaches; I've had a personal coach for about 10 or 11 years now. They [the board] know it; it's not anything I hide at all and [the coach is] somebody who helps me see things that I can't see because I've got biases, I've got blind spots. This is somebody outside the organization; the coach I'm using now, I've used for about two and a half years. He does not have a healthcare background and doesn't even live in Illinois. I work with him weekly on issues, and periodically he comes into town and we spend more concentrated time together. The best way to describe coaching the way that I use it is when you think of a human eye, it cannot look at itself. You can't take the eye out of the eye socket, turn it around, and point it back at yourself and look at yourself. You just can't do that. The coach is that objective person who listens very profoundly to what is being said and then is simply a mirror in feeding back. So I can see things that I wouldn't otherwise be able to see. Coaches don't provide advice; they don't reach into their bag of experience and say, 'I think you ought to do this.' What they do is they continually feed back what they're hearing and allow you to find your own path for resolution on whatever the issue happens to be. That's why this person without a healthcare background can do profound coaching, because [he's] really what I refer to as a contextual coach as opposed to a content coach. They [coaches] don't have to know the details of the content of the issue at hand, but they understand context.

Don also receives informal feedback from Health Insights, a group he helped found 20 years ago. The group is composed of 30 colleagues and is a think tank that convenes twice a year. This group also serves to offer him personal development and career planning advice.

Don's salary is tied to his achievement of corporate objectives and his scores on his performance appraisal. To ensure that competitive salaries are paid, the board hires an outside consulting firm to evaluate CEO salaries and benefits every year. His incentive is based on achievement of corporatewide objectives. In general, Don feels that his evaluation is fair. More generally, in the future, he expects the evaluation needs to include more attention to clinical quality:

> If there is a growing edge in my own review where I think I should be held more accountable, and I think the Executive Committee would be willing to hold me more accountable, it is in the area of clinical quality. I think that is probably a void nationally; I can't say universally that that's a problem. But I think coming into the next five to ten years, whether it's the result of the Leapfrog Group or major payers demanding more around proving and improving quality, I think there's got to be a component of that accountability that the CEO is judged by. So that is a growing edge in our review process and one that I would really welcome as we go forward.

Structurally, there is a problem in Don's evaluation. Because of the short time a board chair is in his position, Don feels that his real contributions are not able to be fully recognized:

> The downside is that they [board chairs] are not there long enough to sink their teeth into our business to a level where they can do a really meaningful job of reviewing the CEO.... It's not even that it's unfair like they don't appreciate what I as CEO or any CEO has done. It's they can't possibly know the business well enough, and because they don't live inside the organization day to day, they can't observe performance. What they can observe is board meetings, board committee meetings, some educational events that you might have for your board and medical staff leadership [and others], but not the day-to-day performance of the CEO. So they're at a disadvantage to do a really rigorous review of the CEO. And I think that comes with volunteer governance in this country. It's the condition we find ourselves in.
>
> Because of volunteer governance, the nature of our businesses, and the fact that chairmen aren't full time in the organization, the quality of the review process is largely left up to the CEO. I won't say totally controlled by the CEO, but if CEOs wanted a superficial review, I think they can probably get that. If they want an in-depth, really constructive, positive review that is going to help them grow and stretch and perform better or refocus their energy on certain things, I think [CEOs] can make that happen if they create that context and ask for it and support the development of a process that will drive out those kinds of competencies. So the review and the process is only going to be as useful for the CEO and the organization as the CEO wants to make it.

In particular, the last two years have been the best reviews in my career because of this process whose design was led by me and my board chairs; that is, each year we've built on it it's gotten better, more meaningful, more focused, and I think more constructive for me as the CEO.

Don's advice to boards seeking to improve their CEO evaluations is to recognize that a good evaluation is premised on the relationship between the board and the CEO:

> If the context for the review is, 'we want to review you in a way that allows us to demonstrate how committed we are to you and your success and the success of the organization,' . . . then there's a lot of feedback that people are willing to receive.

Thus, Don thinks that a board can make almost any kind of comment to the CEO and it will be accepted if the CEO believes that the board is seeking to improve the workings of the hospital and to help the CEO lead the organization. It all comes down to having a trusting relationship:

> If the board doesn't communicate that to the CEO successfully, then any comments about performance, for example 'we don't think you're focusing on the right things,' or 'we'd like more emphasis here,' or 'this was a major problem this year,' will be a cause for concern. If the context is, 'they don't trust me, they're not pleased with my performance, maybe I'm going to lose my job…' [then] you kind of hunker down, you crawl under the table, you don't want to be in those conversations. So the context is decisive. If there's any message that I would communicate to the boards it would be that if it's a context of 'we're committed to your success and the success of the organization and we're going to provide you with feedback so that you can be successful,' [then] I think that will go a long way toward having a really constructive process.

Case Study 2.7

Organization: Overlake Hospital Medical Center, Bellevue, Washington
President/CEO: Kenneth D. Graham, FACHE
Size: 257 beds
Community Profile: Overlake Hospital is a 257-bed not-for-profit free-standing hospital with a foundation, 5 medical clinics, and a venture center designed to generate capital. The hospital is located on the east side

of Lake Washington in what used to be a bedroom community of Seattle but now rivals Seattle as a source of employment with many successful technology firms. The hospital's service area consists of more than 200,000 people within five miles of the hospital. Fifty-two languages are spoken within the community.

Sources of Revenue: 36 percent Medicare, 4 percent Medicaid, 2 percent commercial insurance, 54 percent HMO/managed care, 3 percent self-pay

The evaluation form used in Overlake Hospital was developed in the early 1990s by the board's then Compensation Committee. Since that time, that committee has been renamed the Governance and Management Effectiveness Committee, which is concerned with board continuity, structure, and education as well as review of the CEO. Ken Graham, FACHE, reports that his role as CEO has recently been changed through the addition of a newly hired chief operating officer. As a result, the CEO evaluation form was revised to reflect his expanded role in fundraising.

The chair of the Governance and Management Effectiveness committee is given the main responsibility of coordinating Ken's evaluation. The committee has five members and is designed so that members have long tenure to allow them to see changes over time. The board chair is an ex officio member of the committee. The evaluation is organized by an outside psychological consulting group, the Brighton Group. Brighton collects responses from the 18 board members and from Ken's 6 direct reports. The ten-page document that Brighton provides to the committee includes the following:

1. Introduction, including the number of responses
2. Review of ratings (range 1 to 3) for the current year and two prior years on each section of the questionnaire
3. Comparison between the CEO's self-evaluation and his evaluators
4. Comments on the results—for example, what the board rated highest and lowest and what the vice presidents rated highest and lowest
5. Qualitative comments provided by respondents on the CEO's strengths and weaknesses (growth areas)
6. Review of the three top business priorities—that is, Ken's goals for the past and upcoming years

This report provides the basis of a conversation between Ken, the committee chair, and the board chair; the conversation then yields agreement for the upcoming year's goals. Because the committee meets quarterly, Ken often provides an informal update about the achievement of the current year's goals. However, goals are never altered mid-year. Achieving the goals affects incentive pay only (the opportunity is up to 30 percent of base). The goals are allocated as follows: hospital goals (which are the same for the entire management team) are 60 percent and personal goals are 40 percent.

Specifically, the hospital's goals for the year this interview was conducted involved financial performance measures (i.e., increasing operating margin, limiting capital expenditures, and adding to reserves from operations), which had a 50 percent weight. In addition, 12.5 percent was attached to each of the following four criteria: (1) clinical and organizational quality (i.e., structured patient care improvements, Leapfrog Group goals, and homeland security), (2) employee relations (i.e., turnover, management competencies), (3) physician relations and processes (i.e., conflict identification), and (4) strategic development (i.e., having a plan in place by March 30, obtaining CON [certificate of need] approval for new beds). Ken's personal goals included items such as establishing a leadership council, achieving budget targets for the various entities of the organization, developing a constructive relationship with the neighboring medical center, and fundraising.

In practice, Ken proposes these various corporate and personal goals. The committee sometimes emphasizes one or more and deemphasizes others. In fact, the board reserves the right to simply emphasize one goal over the others. Ken's salary is determined annually by the committee by averaging results of three national salary surveys conducted by the HayGroup, Mercer, and Watson Wyatt. The target for the CEO's pay is the 65th percentile because CEOs earn somewhat higher salaries on the West Coast and in urban areas.

Although physicians are not specifically singled out to evaluate Ken, their impact is represented by the three active physicians and one retired physician on the board. A medical staff satisfaction survey is conducted every three years, but the result of this survey is represented only indirectly in the CEO's appraisal as one item on the evaluation form. Ken considers himself fortunate to have some top corporate executives from billion-dollar companies serving on his Evaluation Committee. They are rational and undaunted by the sometimes large dollar sums discussed.

The evaluation will change in the future. The fiscal year for the hospital is changing so that evaluations that used to be completed between Thanksgiving and Christmas will be completed in August or September. Ken feels that the 360-degree aspect of the process is flawed because not everyone (i.e., board members and Ken's management team) answers the questionnaire. Moreover, the response categories only provide for three levels: (1) does not contribute fully in this area, (2) fully competent contributor in this area, and (3) above and beyond (value added) contributor in this area. Ken's view is that more of a corporate-like evaluation form, perhaps with a larger range of responses permitted with possibly up to seven categories, is likely in the future.

Currently, a financial trigger authorizes the implementation of the incentive compensation program. The policy is that the hospital must achieve 80 percent of its bottom-line budget for the CEO to receive any portion of the incentive opportunity. Looking forward, Ken expects that in the future the form will include more defined measures on whether or not a goal was met, especially financial measures such as profitability and fundraising that show how he is able to adjust to fewer sources of funds:

> This process will probably become more like a corporate evaluation. I don't know exactly how to describe that, but some of the people who are going to work on this in the next six months are used to having a for-profit company's point of view and so there will perhaps be some aspects coming from that direction. . . . It'll tend to be more driven by indicators of organizational vitality, not just that we processed smoothly. A lot of old evaluations asked, 'Did everything go smoothly this year?' I think there's going to be more emphasis on things like profitability and share growth and financial ratios. . . . If you go back to 1993, we didn't have the challenges of not having capital reimbursed by the federal government, [and] we didn't have the challenges of capital formation. We simply had more sources of money than nowadays. We were more profitable, we could make profit, we could negotiate for capital pass-throughs, we could do those kinds of things. Nowadays there's very little sympathy for any of that—you have to earn it the old-fashioned way. If you've got a profit you can support projects with cash or debt financing—great.

Ken offers the following advice to boards who want to improve their CEO's evaluation:

Being proactive and prospective is key—getting the goals and expectations set early and setting up a process that is real. The board should guide the CEO in regards to concerns about vision, focus, and communication. The issues that are harder to talk about are the ones that sometimes need the most attention when it comes down to retention.

Two areas of the evaluation deserve further discussion: homeland security and community health. Ken showed some foresightedness in late 2001 by developing responses to homeland security as one of his clinical and organizational quality objectives. Specifically, the objective states: "Position Overlake as an authoritative leader in homeland security for the East side by June 30, 2002." According to Ken,

> We're working with the fire department, public health department, and the Red Cross. We're putting on seminars together for the Chamber of Commerce and we're putting on focused information sessions with the Red Cross as the convener. We found that before September 11, CEOs were ridiculed if they were too authoritarian. And afterward, everyone expected them to be paternal—you know, 'How do you open the mail, boss?' So now, we're trying to broaden our thinking so that people will look to the hospital as being a real resource in regard to homeland security.

When asked about community health as an objective, Ken states,

> The closest thing we have right now is the homeland security objective and being prepared. We belong to the Partners for a Healthy Community group here, where 5 health systems relate to 100 agencies that coordinate and deploy programs for the community. We work on breast health, family violence, childhood development, and violence prevention. We do our part, but it hasn't risen to a point of being a subject of focused evaluation. The board is looking to me to pull the levers that will move the hospital significantly forward. Developing programs and services for the community is certainly part of my work—ultimately, that's why we're here.

CHAPTER THREE

Evaluating the CEO of the Investor-Owned Hospital

A S ILLUSTRATED IN Chapter 1, investor-owned hospitals in this survey are most likely to provide their CEOs with preestablished written criteria for evaluation. Ninety-four percent of these CEOS said they have preestablished criteria, compared to 76 percent of CEOs in not-for-profit hospitals and 64 percent of CEOs in government hospitals.

In terms of the accountabilities that CEOs are evaluated on, investor-owned CEOs are not significantly different from CEOs in other ownership types. However, even though the results are not statistically significant (probably because of the small number of investor-owned hospital CEO respondents), 9 percent of investor-owned CEOs said they are evaluated on instituting processes to improve community health status. In contrast, 24 percent of government and 28 percent of not-for-profit hospital CEOs said that they are evaluated on such processes. In the case studies below, both CEOs of the investor-owned hospitals we interviewed stated that they are involved with numerous and significant community outreach efforts.

The other notable feature of investor-owned CEO accountabilities is that apparently a higher proportion of them are evaluated on using ethical methods to achieve their goals. Forty-one percent said that this ethical criterion is included in their evaluation, compared to 27 percent of not-for-profit hospital CEOs and 28 percent of government-hospital CEOs.

CASE STUDIES

Following are two case studies based on interviews with the CEO of a small, 70-bed facility in rural Vermont and with the CEO of a 200-bed hospital in Las Vegas, Nevada. Both hospitals are members of large systems. Note that details in the case studies were accurate as of the writing of this monograph; they may have changed in the interim.

Case Study 3.1

Organization: Northwestern Medical Center, Inc., St. Albans, Vermont
CEO: Peter A. Hofstetter, FACHE
Size: 70 beds
Community Profile: Northwestern Medical Center has 70 beds, and its service area has 48,000 people. Agriculture is the primary industry in the area, but other industries call it home, including Ben and Jerry's Ice Cream; Barry Callebaut, USA (a chocolate factory); Peerless Clothing, Inc.; IBM; and the U.S. Immigration and Naturalization Service. The community is 30 miles away from the city of Burlington. Describing the area, the CEO says, "It's pretty rural. If you've been to Montreal through Vermont, you've passed through St. Albans."
Sources of Revenue: 55 percent Medicare, 15 percent Medicaid, 25 percent commercial insurance, 5 percent self-pay

Peter Hofstetter, FACHE, has been with Quorum Health Resources for 18 years. He has been the CEO of Northwestern, a Quorum hospital, for eight years. For his evaluation, Peter completes a self-evaluation form that is also completed by his group vice president (GVP) and the Executive Committee of the board. Peter meets first with the GVP; after that, he meets with the Executive Committee, which is composed of four board officers. The board has 11 members, including medical staff members (two medical staff members are elected, and the president of the medical staff is appointed to the board). The GVP meets in executive session with the Executive Committee; this meeting is where Peter's evaluation is discussed before the results are shared with Peter himself. Thus, Peter really has two bosses; the GVP acts as a facilitator to the entire evaluation process.

The objectives are developed by Peter and approved by the GVP and the board. The evaluation form has three parts:

1. *Goals.* This includes the following:
   a. Management Action Plan, which Peter develops based on the strategic plan. Peter created a grid to show each objective, the standard, and the outcome for the year (see Appendix B.) The plan is approved by the board and can be modified over the year.
   b. Management results, which include items on how the hospital is run such as staffing, motivating, and resolving conflict.
   c. Process indicators, which focus on how the CEO approaches his or her work.
   d. External environmental effects, which weigh items such as if the hospital loses a major admitter, how will it affect how the CEO achieves his or her objectives.

2. *Competency Profile.* This is a list of 35 traits and competencies (e.g., operations, marketing, strategy) against which the CEO is evaluated on the range of 1 (not effective) to 5 (extremely effective).

3. *Development Plan.* This includes future goals within Quorum and continuing education plans.

The CEO is not given a 360-degree evaluation.

Northwestern Medical has no incentive compensation program. However, it gives an arbitrary bonus to the CEO based on the hospital's financial condition; Peter has been given a bonus for the last three to five years. Salary is determined by two mechanisms: (1) Quorum presents the board with ranges based on its internal salary structure, which is related to industry surveys, and (2) the CEO's (and other senior managers') salary increases are about 1 to 1.5 percent above those that the entire staff receives. Peter does not have an employment contract.

For financial measures, Peter uses the national benchmarks that Quorum provides and consults with the Vermont Hospital Association. Also, productivity benchmarks are provided by Premier through its contract with Quorum's 186 hospitals. Peter does very well on all of these indicators: "I think these indicators are interesting. There's more gray stuff these days than there is black and white stuff."

Peter first completes the Competency Profile part of the form; afterward, the GVP and then the board get their chance; the three results are then merged. The profile includes 35 measures. Peter looks for general consistency in responses to these items from all parties. Community health efforts are currently included in the Management Action

Plan. Because the hospital has been doing well financially and is a sole community provider, it has a number of outreach programs, including rural health clinics, prenatal care, smoking cessation, and wellness programs.

The Development Plan part of the form is for Quorum and perhaps can be used with the board as well. The board would want to know whether the CEO has plans to leave. Peter tries to go to an educational program once a year or every other year and to other local presentations. The board tries to make sure he keeps up with continuing education; it was supportive when Peter recertified as a Fellow of ACHE. Peter uses the Position Objectives Form of the evaluation tool to state his overall objectives (left column), specify the expected outcome (middle column), and indicate the actual results (right column). Peter says this of the form: "It's pretty nice because it's clear. This is not the best evaluation in the world but it's pretty functional."

Overall, Peter feels that the evaluation system is fair: "In theory, they could go to my GVP and pull me from the hospital at any time." The big current question is whether the de facto incentive system should become a regular part of the compensation scheme. Emotionally, Peter would like to have this happen, but he knows it would be a difficult conversation to conduct with the board at this time.

The board's self-evaluation follows the CEO's very loosely. It uses the strategic plan, input from the CEO's evaluation, financial issues, planning, board committees, and other factors. Every couple of years, Peter asks the board if it wants to take a look at another self-evaluation form; so far, the board is satisfied with the current form. Each board member completes his or her own self-evaluation, and the results are tabulated and aggregated by the planning committee and then reported to the whole board.

Regarding evaluation changes in the future, Peter states,

> I guess I would like to see it be as much of a two-way street as it could be instead of just going rote through a list of things. I think there will be a lot of issues about staffing in general, and long-term financial issues will continue to be an issue. I have a board that is very interested in what our costs are just as sources of revenue shrink. I would guess there will be more questions about how politically active the hospital would be—both at the state and federal levels.

Peter's advice to boards is as follows:

> Make sure that you and the CEO are talking to each other about the evaluation—that it's not done in a vacuum. I found in small hospitals that it's important that we're all on the same sheet of music and that it be as interactive a process as it can be.

Case Study 3.2

Organization: MountainView Hospital, Las Vegas, Nevada
President/CEO: Mark J. Howard, FACHE
Size: 200 beds
Community Profile: MountainView has 200 beds and provides a full array of services, including neurology and open heart surgery. The hospital has 1,208 physicians on staff, 900 full-time employees, and 1,300 full-time equivalents. In 2001, its budget was $360 million. MountainView's primary service area is the northwest section of Las Vegas, which has a population of 250,000. Besides the gaming industry, bank card processing has been growing as a major source of employment in the area.
Sources of Revenue: 36 percent Medicare, 3 percent Medicaid, 56 percent commercial insurance, 5 percent self-pay

As the CEO of an investor-owned hospital, Mark Howard, FACHE, reports to a market president who represents HCA, the system that owns MountainView, and to a local board. The board evaluates the CEO on seven areas, and the specific measures in these areas are modified from year to year. Mark views quality as the only attribute on which any hospital can market itself. The following are the stakeholders that influence his evaluation:

1. Community, including patients and the press
2. Employers (measured through an annual Gallup survey)
3. Medical staff (measured through an annual survey)
4. Board
5. Corporate office

Meeting financial goals, which is needed for hospital survival, also affects Mark's evaluation. Mark then asks the question of how these six factors affect quality improvement in the hospital.

Mark's immediate supervisor, HCA's divisional market president, gives him 12 goals then selects 5 that are key. These five goals always revolve around the following: quality, physician relations, employees, customers, and finance. The other seven might include other objectives like days in receivables, JCAHO compliance, and bad debt. These goals are woven into the discussion of competencies. At the time of our interview, Mark's goals included 100 percent conformity to the corporate compliance program, building a medical office building, and implementing open heart services. The market president gave him the following items for which to achieve targeted numbers:

1. EBITDA (earnings before interest, taxes, depreciation, and amortization)
2. Employees per occupied bed
3. Satisfaction scores given by physicians
4. Satisfaction scores given by community members
5. Satisfaction scores given by employees

No actual documentation is required to show that these objectives have been met. The same CEO evaluation form is used for all 180 hospitals owned by HCA. The form provides a benchmark for each individual facility and CEO.

Mark's objectives affect only his incentive pay, which is based on achieving financial objectives (50 percent) and satisfaction and quality measures (50 percent). His salary is determined by the movement of the Consumer Price Index; in 2001, CEOs received a 4.5 percent increase. HCA now has the philosophy that CEOs should have a fairly lengthy tenure to prevent a short-term management approach.

Once the CEO completes his own self-evaluation (the other 11 members of the board evaluate him as well), the entire board discusses with him the aggregate performance review. This review is then given to the market president, who sets the CEO's salary for the coming year. (The board does not set salary but helps select the CEO.) Goals are then established by HCA, and prior goals are evaluated. The bonus opportunity is 10 percent of pay, but the real financial opportunity is the stock options that might be offered based on fulfillment of objectives. These options are structured so that the CEO must wait one year to exercise them; only a quarter of each option can be exercised in each of the following four years.

Mark feels that his current evaluation takes into account more stake-holders (see the list of stakeholders above) than at anywhere else he has worked, including the government and not-for-profit sectors. When asked if he considers the involvement of all employees and patients (in addition to the board and medical staff) in his review as a 360-degree evaluation, Mark states,

> Yes, I think it is very much so.... In the medical staff evaluation, they ask, 'How is the administrator running the hospital?' Very few admin-istrators have the medical staff evaluate them. Even on the employee survey, a similar statement is there, 'How is the hospital being managed by the administrator?' So instead of just a few department heads sitting down and saying it's a 360, you've got every employee in the hospital with the opportunity. To me, it's a large 360. The big one is the Gallup poll patient satisfaction survey. One out of four patients in the hospital and one out of eight outpatients are called by the Gallup poll and asked, 'How was your care, the service? Would you come back, do you trust the hospital, what is your loyalty to it?' But patients don't evaluate me; it's the hospital.... So 50 percent of my evaluation is on financials, but the other 50 percent is to see what's happening in these other areas....
>
> In the past, we have not allowed some of our stakeholders, like the employees and the physicians, to have enough say, and I think that's the true indicator of how somebody's doing. I wonder how [some CEOs] get their positions. I think it's because they've had very close rapport with the board chairman and you know, they feed the board chairmen what they want. Well... when our Gallup poll surveys come back, we share it with everybody; even the Medical Executive Committee gets a copy. In our case, we do extremely well for inpatient surgery and tests, but our emergency center just struggles. But at my previous position, we never shared this information; we kept it close to our chests. They wouldn't want anything shared with the employees or the physicians. I think [this system] lets the administrator know how he's doing.
>
> And you know when I talk to the students, I always tell them you have to do these five things. I have seen administrators fired because of the lack of community support, lack of employee support, lack of physician support, lack of board support, lack of corporate office support. So many times we can just get hung up on one area.

To get a real sense of employee morale, Mark arrives in the office most days at 5:30 a.m.; this helps him get to know the night shift. He routinely walks through the hospital to gauge the climate and to see if it has a positive atmosphere. In a strong union city, the unions have failed to penetrate his hospital despite having tried seven times.

Mark foresees that the CEO evaluation form will change in the future to include the bioterrorism issue. But he thinks the current process will likely continue, whereby he meets with the market president monthly (with the employee, patient, physician, and board evaluations in hand) and with his full board every other month. Mark's board's Executive Committee will continue to meet with the medical staff's Executive Committee on the months that he is not meeting with the board. In addition, Mark expects that influencing legislation at the state capitol will continue and that his local board will expect him to continue to work to educate the community about public health and safety issues. In fact, MountainView participates in many community-health-related activities, including holding health fairs, inspecting infant car seats and replacing defective ones for free, conducting bike safety checks and giving away bike helmets, providing labor costs to help immunize the community against influenza and administer childhood vaccinations, and offering space and nurse support to the community for skin care in the summer season.

Mark's advice to boards seeking to improve their CEO's evaluation is as follows:

> I think they [boards] have to be more demanding of the administrators. I think they have to give them greater responsibility—the stewardship type of thing. Too many times in the past, they've said, 'Good bottom line—good year.' What are they doing overall to build it? I've always said good recruiters recruit, but good organizations retain. What's happening with retention? What's happening with turnover? What's happening with the employees? Do you have union issues in the hospital? How are you doing compared to others in your class? I think most hospitals have some type of satisfaction survey. And then you hit the medical staff. What is their satisfaction? How are you coming on discipline? You have to benchmark with others like yourself. I don't think the boards are tough enough.

CHAPTER FOUR

Evaluating the CEO of the Government Hospital

A S INDICATED IN Chapter 1, fewer governmental hospitals (64 percent specifically) use preestablished written criteria for their CEO's evaluation than do not-for-profit or investor-owned hospitals. The case studies in this chapter feature two hospitals that evaluate their CEOs based on preestablished written criteria and one hospital that instead relies on the method of having its CEO prepare a lengthy and comprehensive report on his annual accomplishments.

According to our survey, government hospitals are more likely than not-for-profit and investor-owned hospitals to evaluate their CEOs on leadership ability and on promoting the hospital (e.g., having an effective communication and public relations program). Being direct recipients of tax revenues, these hospitals logically need to communicate to their constituency. As shown in case study 4.1, even the CEO of a small district hospital observed that communications in all forms was the highest priority given to her by the board in her first full year on the job. On the other hand, CEOs in government hospitals are least likely to be evaluated on customer satisfaction, with only about three quarters of these CEOs saying that this item is a factor, compared to more than 90 percent of CEOs in the not-for-profit and investor-owned hospitals who counted on it. The reason for the exclusion of the customer satisfaction criterion may be that government hospitals are often the safety net providers, called on to care for indigent patients using the most economical methods. This may preclude some amenities that contribute to patient satisfaction; realizing this fact, boards or senior officials of government hospitals may be loathe to evaluate CEOS on this criterion.

The survey also suggests that government hospital CEOS are not more likely than others to be evaluated on implementing processes to improve community health or outcomes. But as illustrated in case study 4.2, community health outcomes are a major part of the evaluation of the medical center director of a Veterans Administration (VA) system. In the area of professional role fulfillment, which calls for the CEO to represent the profession to civic and other organizations in the community, government CEOS are more likely to be evaluated than are not-for-profit and investor-owned CEOS. This criterion can be seen as the individual-level counterpart to the institutional-level area of promoting the hospital.

Two other findings about CEOS of government hospitals deserve repeating. First, the compensation of fewer government CEOS (than those in not-for-profit and investor-owned hospitals) is affected by their evaluation; in cases when compensation is affected, it involves either the salary or the bonus but not both. Second, a significantly lower proportion of government hospital CEOS (than the proportion of CEOS in not-for-profit and investor-owned hospitals) feel their evaluation is fair. In separate analyses, we learned that this perception is related to the absence of preestablished written criteria. At Yuma District Hospital, the CEO's evaluation criteria are unilaterally developed and utilized by the board. In the VA system, the medical center director reveals that during the initial period of developing a standardized evaluation form for his review, too many measures were subject to evaluation, a deficiency that was later corrected by the VA's central office. Chesapeake Hospital's CEO also laments the lack of written criteria and rigorous feedback from his board.

CASE STUDIES

Three government hospital case studies are presented in this chapter, starting with a small district hospital in rural Colorado, followed by a VA facility in upstate New York, and concluding with a large hospital along Virginia's eastern seaboard. Note that details in the case studies were accurate as of the writing of this monograph; they may have changed in the interim.

Case Study 4.1

Organization: Yuma District Hospital, Yuma, Colorado
CEO/Executive Vice President: Shana G. Jones, Ph.D., CHE
Size: 11 beds
Community Profile: Yuma District Hospital has 11 staffed beds and is licensed for 23 beds. In addition to its inpatient unit, the hospital has an attached rural health clinic, a home health agency (the only one in two counties), and a Level-IV trauma center. A considerable amount of outpatient surgery at the hospital is provided by surgeons who come from nearby large cities. The hospital has an annual revenue of $9 million, about $500,000 of which is obtained from tax revenue. The community of Yuma consists of 3,500 residents, reflecting a 9 percent increase since the last census; however, its service area has 10,000 people. The area's main industry is agriculture, boasting large hog farms; it also is a major beef producer. Over the past few years, the population has become more ethnically diverse.
Sources of Revenue: 48 percent Medicare; 4 percent Medicaid, 38 percent commercial insurance, 6 percent self-pay

Shana Jones, CHE, took the CEO position at Yuma District Hospital several years ago. When she arrived, she was presented with a list of goals that the board had developed. She was surprised at that, but she acquiesced and managed to accomplish all of them (one goal was deferred). Poudre Valley Health System is the parent company of the hospital and is Shana's employer. Although Shana is in the system's employ, she reports to the hospital board, five members of which are responsible for evaluating her and have the authority to extend her contract. In addition, the board has the authority to make changes to the evaluation criteria during the year.

Along with the list of goals, the board also handed Shana two instruments developed by a consulting firm. The first instrument, "Annual Competency Skills Assessment," is designed to determine the CEO's ability to accomplish tasks in various areas. It has to be completed by the CEO about two months prior to the actual performance review. The CEO uses the instrument to recount her accomplishments during the preceding year. Areas of competency include communications systems; overall operations of the facility; budgeting; performance in any emergency/disaster situation; methods used in confronting issues; corporate goals; community access to care; negotiation skills in acquisitions; working relationships with other executives, medical staff, employees, the board, and the public; regulations and accrediting standards; professional growth activities; civic involvement; performance improvement (required by JCAHO); and cultural factors. After reading the responses of the CEO to each competency area, each board member evaluates the CEO on the 55 questions on the instrument. Then, as a group, the board provides a summary of areas that require improvement. The actual scores are not given to the CEO.

The second instrument includes a position description of about 75 words followed by 12 competencies that reflect the areas in the first instrument. The CEO is evaluated according to three levels: exceeds the standard, meets the standard, and needs improvement. Goals that are set in the previous year are evaluated at the same time as new goals for the coming year are established. These goals are agreed on jointly by the board and the CEO.

Together, both instruments make up the evaluation form that is signed and returned to the CEO. Shana offers further explanation:

> Actually, all our pieces came from Medical Consultants Network, which does the same packet for almost every position there is in healthcare. We thought it was a really nice template because it really did go over all of the different areas with which we got involved. The competency is to verify that you are able to do all those things, the job description is obviously the expectation that you will do those things, and the evaluation is the third piece. The board used the results of the competency and the evaluation form to do my evaluation.

The board increases the salary (bonuses are not paid) using the American Hospital Association's (AHA) survey of compensation as the benchmark. For example, in 2000, the salary was increased by 6.3 percent. The evaluation takes place in October, fortunately just after the annual publication of AHA's compensation survey results.

Shana thinks the criteria are appropriate and measured reasonably. One of the competencies deals with cultural factors, about which Shana states the following:

> I think what they're looking for—at least that's what I did this year—is that our culture at the hospital (for lack of a better term) is somewhat

family oriented. What I gave them was what we had done to enhance that culture and where we were looking to make changes in the employee base. Not so much diversity, but in some cases it's gotten to be a somewhat 'me' environment as opposed to what's best for our community, so there are some cultural-philosophical changes we need to make. It's more based on that, [it's] sort of the mission-driven piece.

Another competency measured is communications systems, to which Shana states the following:

This is my first evaluation here. What we had done in the last year is we went through a computer conversion; we've gone from having no information systems personnel to having a full time information systems CIO. We're in the process of putting in a computer network, which we didn't have in the past. We don't have an intranet; we're obviously able to use the Internet. It's those kinds of things I would talk about. Then, we obviously have a paging system, a phone system, and we have a number of different communication mechanisms.

Many of the goals for Shana's evaluation use the benchmarks published by authorities such as the HARA (Hospital Accounts Receivable Analysis) for accounts receivable, the MGMA (Medical Group Management Association) for clinic days, and so forth.

Although she does not go through a 360-degree appraisal, Shana asks her vice presidents to evaluate her as a manager during their own evaluation. She then shares their individual responses with the board. Because one of the four employed primary care physicians on staff is the medical staff president and serves on the board ex officio, physicians' appraisals are communicated through him.

Shana indicates that some of her goals may be used by the board for its own self-evaluation; however, the board's goals are more directly tied to the strategic plan. To assist the board, Shana has shared with them benchmarking information of similar hospitals in the area on 20 indicators gathered by the Colorado Hospital Association. This information helps to set the board's expectations. Moreover, she shares additional reports with the board about cash flow on a monthly basis.

Shana has a three-year contract. She feels that the evaluation is fair because the goals set out by the board are clear and reasonable and she is able to work without restraint. The evaluation process, she thinks, will likely be the same in the future, but the criteria will change, especially as they relate to new services. For example, at the time of this interview the hospital was going to begin to offer radiation oncology treatments to its community so that residents do not have to drive three hours one-way to Denver for a two-minute treatment. Shana's evaluation will likely reflect these goals: "I'm hoping that in the future, I'm going to be judged even more on whether I'm meeting the community needs." In fact, the recently crafted vision statement will likely become the overarching structure for her evaluations.

When asked if community health status will be a part of her evaluation, Shana says,

> I would hope over time that will come into it. We're a highly agricultural community. We have a fairly high incidence of heart disease and diabetes here primarily because we're also a huge beef producer, so there has to be some temperance on what you would normally suggest for community health… because its their industry, you work around those kinds of issues. But I would certainly hope that we could look at that [goal].

She gives the following advice to boards on improving their CEO evaluations:

> I'd say involve the CEO in the process for one thing; I think the second piece is probably look at things incrementally. You can't change the world overnight. Maybe this year it's one piece, and next year it expands until you finally get to a long-term goal. I think the other issue is that our industry is going through so much change, and now everything you read tells you it can't be incremental change, it has to be completely redesigned, it has to be blown up and started over. And that may be true, but don't ask a CEO to take a bottom line of a hospital from losing $20 million a year to [earning] a $100 million a year profit in one year, because it's not going to happen. It needs to be a realistic goal—a stretch, but realistic—and that's why I think they need to be set in conjunction with the CEO, not in a vacuum.

Case Study 4.2

Organization: Syracuse VA Medical Center, Syracuse, New York
Medical Center Director: James Cody, FACHE
Size: 106 beds

Community Profile: The medical center has 106 acute care beds; a 50-bed nursing home; and eight outpatient clinics, two of which are staffed by the VA and six are under contract. The outpatient clinics are dispersed throughout 18 counties. The medical center employs 1,050 staff and has a budget of $115 million. Syracuse has 147,000 people, but the hospital's service area consists of 150,000 veterans; 35,000 people visited one of the VA facilities for healthcare in fiscal year 2002. This central New York state region has experienced some departures of industry, but its real estate values are increasing—a sign that the area may be ripe for revitalization.

Sources of Revenue: 3 percent commercial insurance, 97 percent government-appropriated funding

James Cody, FACHE, provided us a copy of an annual contract developed by a group at VA's central office for all hospitals in the system. The contract was initiated by Dr. Kenneth Kizer, the VA's Under Secretary for Health, in 1995 in an effort to transform the system's focus from inpatient to outpatient care. Dr. Kizer created a vision: "if you want to get better, then you have to measure how you are doing, and if you don't have any specific targets to shoot at, then it's easy to say that you're making progress, but how are you going to prove it? So that's why these contracts came out."

Dr. Kizer decided to give a common contract to the newly established 22 networks (each of which has from 4 to 10 hospitals) in the United States. Each one of the network directors are held to the performance of the measures in the common contract; thus, the contract extends to the VA as a whole. The VA mission in each network is accomplished through the component medical centers within the network. Each medical center has its own director, who reports to the network director. To ensure that all the directors are aligned with the VA's goals, each medical center director also has the same contract. According to James, "the Under Secretary's vision was that he would use this as a progress monitor to see how well the VA was doing in what he called 'the journey for change'."

Initially, the contract focused only on organizational measures. But measuring a network administrator's achievements by way of its organizational focus was infeasible. Therefore, a separate set of criteria was developed that deal with management indicators (see the A series on this system's evaluation form in Appendix B). The B series indicators deal with specific aspects of quality care outcomes that the VA is targeting. Their achievement is indicative of the quality of care being provided.

James reports to a network administrator. The VA central office and the U.S. Congress serve as the board for the medical center. A 360-degree evaluation is conducted at the medical center. Questions are based on the A series indicators of the contract and sent to peers (five other hospital CEOs in his network); supervisor (the network administrator); and subordinates, including the COO (associate director), chief of nursing, and chief of staff. Based on these evaluations an improvement plan is developed. Sometimes the criteria in the contract are modified during the contract year, and at times new criteria are added to the contract. For example, if Congress decides that more needs to be done about Hepatitis C, then that criterion will be added. The approach taken by the medical center director in such circumstances is to measure the situation at baseline and how much it improved by year's end.

In general, James believes the contract works about as well as any performance evaluation system he has encountered. Although it engenders some competition among the hospitals and networks, it also has clearly improved the health of the community. He cites as an example the measures used to ensure primary care encounters with diabetic patients that require checks for pedal pulses; as a result, amputations have decreased by 60 percent over the last three years at this hospital.

James's salary increase and bonus are dependent on his evaluation. The top bonus attainable is $10,000, based on a five-level gradient for a performance rating: outstanding, excellent, fully satisfactory, satisfactory, and needs improvement. Only outstanding and excellent rating levels are eligible for bonus awards.

In the future, James believes the current emphasis on measurement will continue. Moreover, the VA has been cited as the outstanding federal agency for having developed a scorecard. In fact, the contract has served to focus his work:

I think it has definitely focused things. It's very clear what the expectations are for these areas. In the past, the expectations were never that clear. It's clear when you look down and you see what the standards are for Hepatitis C or pneumococcal immunizations. And it's made a big difference in our patients' lives I believe.

In advising boards on how to improve their CEO's evaluation, James offers the following:

> If I assume correctly that you are referring to improving the contract that I am currently held to, my only suggestion for improvement is to not allow the contract to expand back to the earlier versions, wherein there were so many performance measures that [it] was very difficult to apportion priority to each of the measures (i.e., if everything is the number 1 priority, then nothing is). This latest revision is more practical.

Case Study 4.3

Organization: Chesapeake General Hospital, Chesapeake, Virginia
President/CEO: Donald S. Buckley, Ph.D., FACHE
Size: 291 beds
Community Profile: Chesapeake General Hospital is a misnomer because it really is much more. It has 291 staffed beds, but it is approved for 310. Its budget is $320 million, and it has 550 medical staff and 2,400 employees. Besides the hospital, it has a joint venture to run another hospital, three home health agencies, an outpatient center with outpatient surgery, two assisted living centers, four medical office buildings, two wellness centers, and a for-profit personal medical supply company. Chesapeake's primary service area has 372,155 people, and its secondary service area has 1 million and includes residents in four cities—Norfolk, Virginia Beach, Portsmouth, and Chesapeake. Businesses in the area include insurance, management consulting, manufacturing companies with foreign headquarters, a QVC (home shopping network) call center, and a naval shipyard and naval base. Perhaps as many as 250,000 people in the area are connected to the military; some of them are civilian employees who use their CHAMPUS benefits at the hospital.
Sources of Revenue: 41 percent Medicare, 2 percent Medicaid, 24 percent commercial insurance, 22 percent HMO, 6 percent self-pay

Don Buckley, FACHE, used to complete a ten-category evaluation form with questions in each category, but after several years the board discontinued using it. Since 1995, the board has been using a general type of evaluation, requiring Don to provide an oral summary of his activities for the year. Thus, Don prepares a 40 to 50 page document entitled "Evaluation of President/CEO." The document contains the following (see Appendix B):

1. List of Don's responsibilities
2. Financial numbers compared to the previous year. Included here are benchmarks on key indicators and narrative highlighting the outcomes, including some discussion of reserves and a comparison of the system with outside benchmarks.
3. Results of the annual survey of physicians on staff regarding their satisfaction. Included here is a discussion of medical staff needs and a comparison of the current satisfaction data with the previous year's.
4. Patient satisfaction report. A quarterly report is prepared through surveys of discharged patients from inpatient, outpatient, and emergency departments. This information is aggregated for the year.
5. Results of the employee relations survey. The 60 to 70 percent response rate is representative. The survey is conducted by AON, which publishes the national survey of employee commitment. A one-and-a-half page narrative accompanies this section.
6. Quality and cost-enhancement achievements. This section discusses improvements in quality, which are related to benchmarks published by Premier. JCAHO's ONYX system is used to compare these improvements with those of other hospitals. The quality indicators are then related to cost reductions such as reduced length of stay.
7. Community-outreach initiatives. Don's narrative recaps the monthly reports he gives his board concerning outreach, including financial contributions and activities such as screenings conducted, presentations made, and partnerships initiated.
8. Basic goals and objectives. This is a simple recount of the aims set out at the last review and the achievements since then.
9. Other accomplishments. This is a report on activities that were not on the formal to-do list but were nevertheless accomplished, such as opening a new assisted living facility or a fitness center.
10. Status report on activities and projects. This narrative refers to efforts that are underway, such as a joint venture with another hospital.

11. Strategic planning update. This is a two-page narrative on Don's vision, the future of the system, and issues that he thinks need to be addressed.

12. State-of-the-system report. This is a potential stand-alone section that provides a wrap-up of clinical, rehabilitation, administration, and support services. Other outsourced functions, like information technology, are discussed here as well. This section can be used by a visiting consultant who wants to know the issues that the system is currently confronting.

The board reviews Don's statement and, as a group, meets with him to discuss his performance and his raise; currently, the board uses Premier's compensation survey as a guide to determining Don's raise. (He does not receive incentive compensation.) The evaluation is not quantitative; no formula is used to determine the amount of the raise. Instead, it is a subjective assessment of Don's performance. After the evaluation, Don does not have specific guidelines for what he needs to do, as he states:

> When I come out of an evaluation, sometimes I don't have specifics. In other words, they don't say, 'Look, you really need to work on your medical staff relations, or we think you need to spend more time externally.' I don't get that type of feedback. Recently, they said, 'Financially, things are not going the way they have been, but they're not going that way anywhere, but you're doing a great job.' I think that the way we do it, they [the board] get more information and I get less constructive criticism.... What I think would be ideal [is] I would like to continue providing them with this document, but they take each of these sections—for instance, medical staff relations—and provide comments [like] 'Good job in finding out about medical staff needs; would like to have medical staff more involved in operational planning, for example... then go to employee relations, [saying] 'Turnover needs to be reduced; more efforts in creating a pipeline for health careers....' I will be talking to them about that... I'm in my 31st year now.

Don's board has 11 members, 2 of whom are physicians on the medical staff and 2 physicians are ex officio members (the president and president-elect of the medical staff). Board members are political appointees by the city council; they have terms of four years that are renewable. Don does not have a 360-degree evaluation; only the board evaluates him and he doesn't expect to see any big changes with this in the future, but he sees one exception. The medical staff president and the medical staff president-elect may, in the future, want to sit with the board chair and give him feedback about the CEO's performance. Don does not think that his reports should provide this kind of feedback.

Ideally, Don would like the board to have a compensation committee to evaluate the CEO, determine salary, and address succession planning; various consultants have recommended this idea to Don as well. The board should hold evaluations meetings with the CEO three times annually to (1) approve goals, (2) conduct a mid-year review, and (3) to conduct the year-end evaluation. The mid-year review would provide early feedback to the CEO and allow the CEO to discuss progress toward his goals. During this review, the board can address any concerns and suggest improvement.

Don's advice to boards that want to improve their CEO's evaluation is to obtain as much information from the CEO and the medical staff; a small committee of the board, preferably a compensation committee, should be assigned to gather this information. Ideally, boards should provide specific constructive criticism, and praise when necessary, on a regular basis. Evaluation meetings should present no surprises for the CEO; being open at these meetings is critical. The entire board or individual members should voice any concerns to the board chair prior to the evaluation; afterward, the chair should pass these concerns along to the CEO. Here are Don's words:

> One, I think they need a tremendous amount of information from their CEO so that they're informed when they're making their evaluation. Two, they do need input from the medical staff. I don't believe that the board should go to the vice presidents or anybody in management for input. Three, I think that it should be done by a small committee—a compensation committee. Four, I think the compensation committee should meet with the CEO before it goes to the board. Five, I think that the CEO should be given constructive criticism, comments, and compliments that are as specific as possible. I think that it needs to be given on a regular basis.... They [the board] ought to get the material [for evaluation] a month before it is to take place so they are not five or six months late in doing the evaluation.
>
> Now, throughout the year, for instance, I meet with my chairman monthly at least. But there ought to be a sit down with the CEO after

six months for just general comments. I think part of evaluation is open communication throughout the year. Evaluations should not really bring up any surprises. In other words, don't go 12 months and then say, 'Look you're doing a terrible job with the medical staff, you've got one month to improve it.' Just like I do with the vps. I think openness is so important because so often a CEO will call me and say, 'You know, the board's meeting in three hours and is planning to terminate me. I really don't know why this is taking place.'

Open communication starts with the board to the chairman and then to the CEO. The chairman ought to be the pipeline to the CEO. If individual board members start going to the CEO saying, 'I think you ought to start doing this,' well an individual board member has no authority until he's meeting with the group as a whole. And so the group as a whole should communicate to the chairman who then communicates with the CEO.... What is uncomfortable is when there are concerns raised that you don't know about.

CHAPTER FIVE

Lessons Learned and Future Directions

THIS CHAPTER IS a summary of the main CEO evaluation processes that, according to our survey and case study findings, are followed by hospitals today. Here, we identify processes that seem to be working and the directions toward which these processes are headed. Overall, the survey suggested that most hospital CEOs are being evaluated based on preestablished written criteria and that CEO evaluations are conducted annually. Depending on the size of the board, some evaluations are conducted by the whole board while others are performed by a subcommittee of the board or by an official in the health system who is superior to the CEO.

THE PROCESS

Certain elements of the evaluation process differ for each hospital CEO, of course. But the main methods are similar throughout, consisting of the following steps:

1. CEO conducts a self-evaluation
2. (Optional) Board collects evaluations from CEO's direct reports, community liaisons, physicians, and other constituents
3. Board conducts its own evaluation of the CEO
4. Board and CEO (and others if indicated) discuss differences in evaluation and directions for coming year

Other major points indicated by the survey are as follows:

- Only in rare instances are goals that were established at the beginning of the year modified. The reason for the goal modification is when a major change occurs, such as a pending merger or a move by a key group of physician admitters.
- Sometimes goals for the CEO are used by the entire management team.
- Achievement of goals usually affects the CEO's compensation.
- Usually the board's candid and brutal comments are acceptable to the CEO if the CEO perceives the comments to be helpful in making him or her do a better job and thus continue in the leadership role. Boards are advised to provide constructive feedback to their CEO.

THE VALUE OF BENCHMARKING

Many of the hospital CEOs featured in the case studies informed us of their organizations' reliance on benchmark data to compare or base their own performance or practices against those of similar organizations. Here are lessons learned from their experiences:

- By comparing hospital data with similar hospitals, current performance gaps and best practices can be adopted.
- To be fair, benchmarking standards should be adjusted for patient mix and community differences.
- Benchmarking measures are best developed by external agents such as the government (e.g., Centers for Medicare & Medicaid Services); associations (e.g., American Hospital Association, Healthcare Financial Management Association); alliances (e.g., Premier or VHA); investor-owned provider organizations (e.g., HCA, Quorum); or commercial organizations such as Solucient, MECON, CHIP, Press Ganey, or JCAHO.
- Benchmarking can be used for the following three categories of the CEO's evaluation:

    1. *Institutional Success.* These statistical indicators are recommended for use on executive report cards (Devan and Willams 1999):

a. Total expense per case mix index (CMI) weighted adjusted discharge. For example, the board can track the overall performance of the hospital using this indicator. National data show that in 1999, the 25th percentile was $4,041, the 50th percentile was $4,640, and the 75th percentile was $5,448. Such information can be used to provide perspective about an individual hospital's total expense. Through decomposition using other data, this information can also determine the causes of higher than normal expenses, which possibly will lead to reducing these costs.
   b. Labor expense per adjusted discharge
   c. Staffing ratios
   d. Nonlabor expense per adjusted discharge
   e. Gross revenue per adjusted discharge
   f. Net revenue per adjusted discharge
   g. Capital expense per adjusted discharge
   h. Clinical utilization expense per adjusted discharge
   i. Professional fees

2. *Community Health Status*
   a. Processes might include achieving the targeted number of patient visits made to outreach clinics, number of employees involved in community outreach projects, and number of educational programs offered to community members and establishing productive linkages with public health agencies (ACHE 2001).
   b. Outcome indices include infant mortality rate; percentage of low-birthweight babies; teenage birth rate; youth suicide rate; rate of hospitalization for mental illness of children and youth; percentage of adolescent health-risk behaviors such as cigarette use, binge drinking, and marijuana use; incidence of childhood measles; and incidence of traumatic head injuries (Simmes et al. 2000).
   c. Leaders of not-for-profit healthcare organizations are encouraged to link compensation arrangements for their executives to the provision of community benefits (Milstead 1999).

3. *Professional Role Fulfillment*

   a. For continuing education. Hold CEOs accountable for attending a minimum of eight hours of formal continuing education per year. This is the standard used by ACHE for its affiliates.

   b. For representing the profession. Establish a baseline measure of involvement in civic and other community organizations. Then assess whether such involvement continues or grows in subsequent years.

   c. For leadership/mentoring. Determine if the hospital has a formal mentoring program. Then establish a target number of mentor-protégé relationships between senior managers and junior managers or students each year.

   d. For ethical methods to achieve goals. Insist that the CEO abides by the Code of Ethics and the policy statements published by ACHE. Also encourage executives to review ACHE's ethical policy statements and to complete ACHE's Ethical Self-Assessment on an annual basis.

THE VALUE OF 360-DEGREE EVALUATIONS

Obtaining feedback from peers and subordinates, in addition to comments from the board, is becoming common. Table 1.5 shows that over half of the CEOs in the survey felt that their performance should be evaluated by others on the management team. In addition, between 40 and 50 percent of the CEOs thought that physicians on the hospital's medical staff should evaluate them. Moreover, most of the CEOs featured in the case studies stated that their evaluation includes a 360-degree appraisal.

Unfortunately, few studies prove or disprove the value of 360-degree evaluations. At this time, hospitals may wish to experiment with 360s and then decide if they improve the quality and depth of their current evaluation. Certainly, boards have to ensure that subordinates' and peers' reviews are aggregated and reported to the CEO anonymously. One affiliate in our survey stated that his board contracts with an outside agency to collect the opinions of eight senior executives under him and physicians. This information is gathered every other year rather than every year to reduce the time and expense of such assessments.

CONCLUSION

The survey and the 12 in-depth interviews with CEOs demonstrate a great deal of variation in CEO evaluation processes. When compared with our prior research—*Achieving Success Through Community Leadership* (Weil, Bogue, and Morton 2001) and *Rekindling the Flame* (ACHE 2001)—however, we find that hospital boards and those charged with CEO evaluation are opening up the process, expanding the number of people involved in evaluation, looking to external agencies to help them establish benchmarks, and developing routine data-collection forms to facilitate the review process.

CHAPTER SIX

Suggested Criteria for CEO Evaluation

ONSIDERING THE INFORMATION presented in the previous chapters, in this chapter we suggest criteria and measures that boards and corporate officers can use in conducting their hospital CEO's evaluation.

THREE SUBSTANTIVE AREAS

Our survey shows that the three typical areas of substantive evaluation—institutional success, community health status, and professional role fulfillment—are addressed differently in contemporary CEO evaluations. Table 1.1 makes apparent that the accountabilities reflecting institutional success are most often evaluated by the hospitals in the survey. Some accountabilities are used more than others—for example, financial concerns and customer satisfaction are generally more popular than influencing legislation and regulations. Despite these preferences, all accountabilities under institutional success are included in this chapter; individual hospitals can decide whether any should be excluded from their own criteria in this area.

The two accountabilities—community health improvement processes and community health outcomes—that reflect the CEO's involvement in enhancing the area's health status are not commonly used as measures. In fact, in most cases, less than a quarter of CEOs told us that they are evaluated based on these accountabilities. Nevertheless, boards and corporate officers that add these measures to their CEO's evaluation will more closely align the mission of the hospital to the goals of its executives, particularly given the fact that not-for-profit hospitals have to show their contribution to benefit the community. Professional role fulfillment (the third area) is measured using four accountabilities, of which the most commonly used is representing the profession to other organizations. The other accountabilities are considered as well, albeit by a minority of hospitals.

To further understand the use of the above accountabilities in CEO evaluations, we analyzed the evaluation forms actually used by the hospitals presented in the case studies (see Appendix B). Table 6.1 indicates that the forms used by a majority of the hospitals in our interviews include the various accountabilities under institutional success. Few hospitals have forms that include community health status accountabilities, and only a minority of hospitals use forms that measure the four accountabilities of professional role fulfillment. In addition, Table 6.1 shows that a majority of the forms list specific criteria to evaluate the CEO's relationships with the board and the medical staff. Five of the 12 hospitals in the case studies evaluate their CEO based on achieving annual objectives and on teamwork. These relatively subjective measures listed in the majority of the forms can be incorporated into the leadership accountability in the area of institutional success.

Including specific objective benchmarks in evaluating the CEO seems prudent. Boards and corporate officers may wish to consult with one or more of the organizations listed in Chapter 5 (under the section entitled "The Value of Benchmarking") to help them devise suitable benchmarks for their CEO evaluation.

INSTITUTIONAL SUCCESS

Institutional success is the core of the CEO's evaluation. It includes the hospital's ability to deliver healthcare services, maintain financial viability, uphold its reputation, and realize reasonably harmonious relations with physicians and other healthcare organizations. Suggested measures for each accountability under this area are listed below.

1. *Planning.* The CEO participates with the board in charting the course the hospital must take to meet the community's needs. General questions here might include the following:

- Does the CEO play a major role in the long-range or strategic planning process?
- Are clear, easily understood plans that are regularly updated to meet changing conditions in effect?

The CEO pursues the following activities to carry out the planning function:

- evaluates the effects of external forces on the institution;
- recommends long-range plans that support the institution's philosophy and general objectives;
- informs trustees about and interests them in current trends, issues, problems, and activities in healthcare;
- recommends hospital policy positions concerning legislation, government administrative policy, and other public policy matters;
- helps identify potential board members with the necessary expertise to craft informed policy; and
- updates long-range plans.

2. *Human resources management.* The CEO must ensure the attainment of hospital objectives through the selection, development, motivation, evaluation, and retention of hospital personnel. General questions here might include the following:

- Does the hospital recruit adequate numbers of qualified staff to carry out programs and services?
- Are human resources being properly allocated to carry out the mission and goals/objectives of the hospital?
- Is the rate of employee absenteeism and turnover at an acceptable level?
- Are the results of employee attitude surveys generally positive?
- Has low employee performance contributed to excessive costs?

To effect the human resources function, the CEO does the following:

- specifies personnel accountabilities,
- evaluates performance regularly,
- establishes proper departmentalization and delegation,

	Not For Profit							Investor Owned		Government		
	St. John's Lutheran Hospital, Libby, MT	Atlantic General Hospital, Berlin, MD	Keokuk Health Systems, Keokuk, IA	Bay Area Medical Center, Marinette, WI	Wadley Regional Medical Center, Texarkana, TX	Central DuPage Health System, Winfield, IL	Overlake Hospital Medical Center, Bellevue, WA	Northwestern Medical Center, Inc., St. Albans, VT	MountainView Hospital, Las Vegas, NV	Yuma District Hospital, Yuma, CO	Syracuse VA Medical Center, Syracuse, NY	Chesapeake General Hospital, Chesapeake, VA
Institutional Success												
Planning	✓		✓	✓	✓	✓	✓	✓	✓	✓	✓	✓
Human resources management	✓	✓	✓	✓	✓	✓	✓	✓	✓	✓	✓	✓
Quality services	✓	✓	✓	✓	✓	✓	✓	✓	✓	✓	✓	✓
Allocating financial/physical/human resources	✓	✓	✓	✓	✓	✓	✓		✓	✓	✓	✓
Compliance with regulations	✓	✓	✓	✓	✓	✓	✓	✓	✓	✓		
Influencing legislation and regulations									✓			
Promotion of the hospital					✓		✓	✓	✓		✓	
Customer satisfaction		✓		✓	✓	✓		✓	✓	✓	✓	✓
Leadership: communication and succession planning	✓	✓	✓				✓	✓	✓	✓	✓	✓
Community Health Status												
Processes to improve community health		✓			✓		✓		✓			✓
Outcomes to signify improvement					✓	✓						✓
Professional Role Fulfillment												
Continuing professional education	✓				✓						✓	
Representing the profession			✓		✓							
Leadership/mentoring								✓				
Ethical methods to achieve goals									✓			

TABLE 6.1 (continued)

Other Areas of Evaluation	NOT FOR PROFIT							INVESTOR OWNED		GOVERNMENT		
	St. John's Lutheran Hospital, Libby, MT	Atlantic General Hospital, Berlin, MD	Keokuk Health Systems, Keokuk, IA	Bay Area Medical Center, Marinette, WI	Wadley Regional Medical Center, Texarkana, TX	Central DuPage Health System, Winfield, IL	Overlake Hospital Medical Center, Bellevue, WA	Northwestern Medical Center, Inc., St. Albans, VT	MountainView Hospital, Las Vegas, NV	Yuma District Hospital, Yuma, CO	Syracuse VA Medical Center, Syracuse, NY	Chesapeake General Hospital, Chesapeake, VA
Board relations	✓	✓	✓	✓	✓	✓	✓	✓	✓	✓		
Relations with boards of system and member organizations					✓					✓	✓	
Medical staff relations	✓	✓	✓	✓	✓	✓	✓	✓	✓	✓		
Achieves annual objectives				✓	✓	✓	✓		✓	✓		✓
Teamwork: persistence				✓	✓				✓			
delegation				✓	✓				✓			
Decision making					✓			✓		✓		
Sensitive to political issues					✓						✓	

✓ indicates measure is on current CEO evaluation form

Suggested Criteria for CEO Evaluation   73

- participates as teacher and preceptor in educational programs,
- helps prevent occupational mishaps,
- encourages employee retention, and
- promotes high morale.

3. *Quality services.* The CEO monitors the hospital's patient care activities. Through coordination with the board, medical staff, and nursing personnel, the CEO establishes policies needed to ensure high-quality healthcare services. General questions here might include the following:

- Does the CEO establish methods for evaluating patient care activities and are errors appropriately recognized? For example, by addressing why a mistake was made (not only who made the mistake), executives can better identify and address systemic problems.
- Has the hospital adopted a system-oriented approach to medication-error reduction? For example, has the hospital implemented standard procedures for ordering and dispensing medications? Are there special procedures for using high-risk medications?
- Has the CEO attempted to prevent medical errors? For example, has the hospital adopted one or more of the following processes: computerized physician order-entry of medication orders, referring patients in need of high-risk procedures to hospitals that meet a specific annual volume criterion, and establishing round-the-clock coverage of surgical and medical intensive care units by intensivists?
- Are there adequate reporting structures? For example, are surgeons provided feedback about the patients' infection rates? Is the voluntary infection monitoring service by Centers for Disease Control utilized? If the hospital has adopted a continuous quality improvement philosophy, has the CEO acquired feedback for evaluating the hospital's performance in patient care delivery?
- Does the hospital meet the requirements of licensing and accrediting agencies? Are cited deficiencies being addressed in a timely and comprehensive way?

In carrying out the quality accountability, the CEO should take a number of initiatives, including the following:

- ensure institutional operating stability by creating a working environment that is satisfactory to staff and physicians;
- consult with medical, nursing, and other clinical staff concerning the quality of patient care within the hospital;
- consult with leaders of medical, nursing, and other clinical staff prior to establishing new policies; likewise, the CEO ascertains the availability of resources for implementing policies;
- appropriately represent the board to the medical staff;
- coordinate the efforts of the medical staff, board, and management staff in recruiting and retaining medical staff; and
- advocate and implement continuous quality improvement in all hospital systems.

4. *Management of financial, physical, and human resources.* The CEO ensures that healthcare services are produced in a cost-effective manner—that is, efforts are made to employ economies while maintaining an acceptable level of quality. General questions here might include the following:

- Are there effective, understandable operating and capital budgeting processes in place?
- Is the board informed on a regular basis about significant financial matters?
- Are there sufficient financial controls?
- Is the hospital's financial condition routinely audited by an external firm, and are the results reported to the board?
- Is the hospital's operating margin consistent with budgeted expectations?

To effect this accountability, the CEO should pursue the following types of activities:

- ensure the sound fiscal operation of the institution, including the timely, accurate, and comprehensive development of an annual budget and its implementation;

- plan for capital equipment through the budget, and obtain board approval for capital purchases above a specified threshold;
- plan the use of physical resources of the institution;
- obtain adequate insurance policies to protect against damage to the facility, lawsuits, and others;
- arrange contractual relationships with consultants, contractors, architects, and other parties as appropriate on behalf of the board when planning and developing facilities, finances, and personnel programs;
- combine organizational resources in such a way that maximizes, in quantity and quality, a set of results; and
- achieve budget objectives.

5. *Compliance with regulations.* The CEO ensures compliance with regulations governing hospitals and the rules of accrediting bodies by continually monitoring the hospital's facilities, programs, and services and by initiating changes as required. General questions here might include the following:

- Does the CEO share reports from external evaluators with the board?
- Is there a plan to correct deficiencies cited?

To effect this accountability, the CEO should pursue the following types of activities:

- participate as needed in litigation for the hospital, and inform the board of any need to initiate litigation;
- maintain a well-functioning quality assurance program with strong links to the board, and keep the board notified of any hospital-related malpractice claim;
- ensure that the hospital meaningfully participates in licensing and accrediting processes;
- approve final settlements of all lawsuits against the hospital (the board may wish to reserve this power within limits); and
- meet or exceed JCAHO or other accrediting and licensing agency criteria.

6. *Influencing legislation and regulations.* The CEO works with legislators, regulators, and representatives of the healthcare sector to ensure that legislative and regulatory policies promote the health of the community and do not place unmanageable encumbrances on the hospital. General questions here might include the following:

- Does the CEO communicate with the board, hospital staff, and community groups about the expected impact of pending legislation or regulations on the hospital?
- Does the CEO provide needed data and other supporting evidence to spokespersons and other hospital advocates?
- Does the CEO take on a leadership role in local, state, or national forums in representing hospitals and the healthcare needs of the community?

To effect this accountability, the CEO should pursue the following types of activities:

- support national, state, and provincial healthcare associations;
- testify before legislative and regulatory bodies; and
- solicit board and community support for policies that advance healthcare.

7. *Promotion of the hospital.* The CEO encourages the integration of the hospital with the community by establishing an effective communication and public relations program. General questions might include the following:

- Is the CEO well positioned and professionally involved in community healthcare and related activities?
- Is the CEO visible in the community and a good public relations emissary for the hospital?

To effect this accountability, the CEO should pursue the following types of activities:

- solicit feedback from customers on type, availability, and quality of services;

- listen and respond appropriately to the medical staff, employees, and volunteers to improve services and generate community involvement with the hospital;
- speak to community groups concerning health problems and new programs;
- represent the board to the community;
- represent the hospital in state, provincial, and national associations that are concerned with healthcare delivery;
- initiate, develop, and maintain cooperative relationships with the business community and with other hospitals;
- participate in fundraising efforts; and
- achieve goals related to promoting the hospital.

8. *Leadership.* The CEO conceptualizes, transmits, and effects a personal vision of health delivery in the community. By interacting with community leaders, including the board and medical staff, the CEO increases public understanding of health policy issues, the role of the hospital, and needed directions for change. In addition, the CEO (using ethical and equitable methods) articulates a set of values that serves to motivate others in advancing the hospital's programs and services consistent with community need. Through leadership, the CEO acts to avoid crises but manages them decisively and with sensitivity if they occur. General questions here might include the following:

- Does the CEO have a clear vision of the future of the hospital and its contribution to community well-being?
- Does the CEO communicate the vision effectively and motivate others in the community and the hospital to effect this vision?
- Does the CEO prioritize activities to avert crises?
- When crises occur, does the CEO act decisively in a timely way to mitigate adverse consequences?

To effect this accountability, the CEO should pursue the following types of activities:

- envision the hospital's role in providing healthcare to the community in new ways, or enlarge existing services to improve community health;

- stimulate interest in the hospital's programs and services among community members and members of the medical and hospital staff;
- exercise judgment in pursuing the strategic objectives of the hospital by insisting on conforming to ethical guidelines and accepted business mores;
- act to avoid crises and help to overcome them by preparing for them through protocols and decisive action; and
- foster a smoothly functioning, efficient organization through timely and effective resolution of disruptions, and establish a plan for crisis intervention in the event of strikes, disasters, and other issues.

COMMUNITY HEALTH STATUS

The hospital's ultimate reason for being is to improve the health of the community. Therefore, part of the CEO's evaluation appropriately should focus on the community's health status. However, because the hospital is not the only community institution dedicated to improving health, the CEO's evaluation needs to be concerned with only the elements of community health status that he or she can reasonably be expected to influence. General questions in this area might include the following:

- Is the CEO knowledgeable about healthcare needs and trends in the hospital's community?
- Are attempts to address community healthcare needs incorporated into the hospital's strategic plan?

To effect this accountability, the CEO should pursue the following types of activities:

- provide evaluators with data that track key community health outcome indices such as infant mortality rates and the incidence or prevalence of diseases in the community or service area;
- encourage maximum healthcare benefits for community residents, including implementing the hospital's mission statement by assessing the community's overall health status and integrating the

mission and community service responsibilities into the organization's policy development and program planning; and

- articulate a concern for the community throughout the hospital, such as developing initiatives that provide community service, assist in social projects, and advance public dialog on policy issues affecting the community.

PROFESSIONAL ROLE FULFILLMENT

The CEO, as a practicing professional, must stay abreast of contemporary practices in the management and leadership of hospitals. Ideally, the CEO works to advance the profession of healthcare management. General questions in this area might include the following:

- Does the CEO allocate time for his or her continuing professional education?
- Does the CEO contribute to the healthcare management profession by representing it to other groups as well as participating in his or her own professional society's activities?
- Is the CEO willing to share leadership experiences with others?

To effect this accountability, the CEO should pursue the following types of activities:

- maintain his or her professional competence by pursuing educational programs that are meaningful and relevant to effective performance;
- abide by codes of ethics, which are promulgated by leading hospital, trade, and professional associations;
- serve as an articulate spokesperson for the healthcare management profession and work to ensure its development; and
- engage in educational mentoring programs by providing administrative internships or fellowships in the hospital.

CONCLUSION

This chapter is a summary of the central accountabilities by which hospital CEOs should be evaluated. Each hospital has a unique set of strategies that must be addressed to enable it to fulfill its mission. The account-abilities identified are central to many CEOS' roles, helping them form the basis for a management plan. The challenge to individual evaluators is adapting the foregoing accountabilities to the immediate concerns of the hospital so that its leadership team has congruent expectations of the CEO's performance.

References

American College of Healthcare Executives. 2001. *Rekindling the Flame: A Casebook.* Chicago: Health Administration Press. (For an online version of the publication, visit ache.org/PUBS/Research/rekindling.cfm.

Coile, R. C., Jr. 2003. *Futurescan 2003: A Forecast of Healthcare Trends: 2003–2007*, pp. 2–4. Chicago: Health Administration Press.

Cutt, J., and V. Murray. 2000. *Accountability and Effectiveness Evaluation in Non-Profit Organizations.* London: Routledge.

Devan, V. R., and M. Williams. 1999. "Measuring Up: Benchmarking Tools Can Enhance Executive Performance." *Trustee* (May): 6–9.

Milstead, L. 1999. "The Pressure Is On: Tying Executive Pay to Community Benefits." *Health Forum Journal* (March/April): 47–49.

Simmes, D. R., M. R. Blaszcak, P. S. Kurtin, N. L. Bowen, and R. K. Ross. 2000. "Creating a Community Report Card: The San Diego Experience, Carefully Selected Statistics From an Annual Snapshot of Community Health and Well-being." *American Journal of Public Health* 90 (6): 880–82.

Weil, P., A. Richard, J. Bogue, and R. L. Morton. 2001. *Achieving Success Through Community Leadership.* Chicago: Health Administration Press.

RECOMMENDED READINGS

Fielding, J. E., C. E. Sutherland, and N. Hallon. 1999. "Community Health Report Cards: Results of a National Survey." *American Journal of Preventive Medicine* 17 (1): 79–86.

Modern Healthcare. 2001. "100 Top Hospitals: National Benchmarks." *Modern Healthcare* Special Supplement, February 26.

Murphy, E. C. 1996. *Leadership IQ: A Personal Development Process Based on a Scientific Study of a New Generation of Leaders.* New York: John Wiley & Sons, Inc.

Olden, P., and D. Clement. 1998. "Well-Being Revisited: Improving the Health of a Population." *Journal of Healthcare Management* 43 (1): 36–50.

Shwartz, M., A. S. Ash, and L. I. Iezzoni. 1997. "Comparing Outcomes Across Providers." In *Risk Adjustment for Measuring Health Outcomes*, 2nd edition, edited by Lisa I. Iezzoni, 471–516. Chicago: Health Administration Press.

ACHE Fax Survey

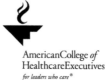

AmericanCollege *of*
HealthcareExecutives
for leaders who care®

Evaluating the Performance of the Hospital CEO

This fax survey focuses on hospital CEO performance evaluations. Please take 5–10 minutes to answer the following questions. All information you provide will be strictly confidential. Individual respondents will not be identified in any reports without their consent. Results will be published in the Winter 2002 issue of *Chief Executive Officer* and will be used to update ACHE's monograph on hospital CEO evaluation.

1. How many beds are staffed for use at your hospital?

> 500+...1
> 350–499..2
> 200–349..3
> 100–199..4
> Less than 100.....................................5

2. What is the ownership status of your hospital?

> Investor-owned...........................1
> Religiously-sponsored.............2
> Not-for-profit secular..............3
> Government...............................4

3. Is your performance evaluated using pre-established written criteria?

> Yes.......................................1 ———➤ Proceed to question 4.
> No...2 ———➤ Please skip to question 6.

4. If yes, please circle the letters of the criteria that are currently used in your evaluation; for each criterion please list how your performance is measured:

   Institutional Success

   a. Planning (e.g., updating strategic plan)

   How is your performance measured? _____

b. Human resource management (e.g., employee turnover rate)
   How is your performance measured? _____

c. Quality services (e.g., risk-adjusted mortality)
   How is your performance measured?_____

d. Allocating financial, physical, and human resources (e.g., operating surplus)
   How is your performance measured?_____

e. Compliance with regulations (e.g., JCAHO citations)
   How is your performance measured?_____

f. Influencing legislation and regulations (e.g., representing community health needs to legislators)
   How is your performance measured?_____

g. Promotion of the hospital (e.g., publicity campaigns)
   How is your performance measured?_____

h. Customer satisfaction (e.g., patient satisfaction scores)
   How is your performance measured?_____

i. Leadership (e.g., communication, succession planning)
   How is your performance measured?_____

j. Please specify any other criteria used to gauge institutional success.
   _____

Community Health Status

a. Processes to improve community health (e.g., percent of community with flu immunization)
   How is your performance measured?_____

b. Outcomes to signify improved community health (e.g., infant mortality rate in community)
   How is your performance measured? _____

c. Please specify any other criteria regarding improved community health.
   _____

Professional Role Fulfillment

a. Continuing professional education (e.g., hours of off-site training)
   How is your performance measured?_____

b. Representing the profession (e.g., appointments held, including civic organizations)
   How is your performance measured?_____

c. Sharing leadership experiences with others/mentoring (e.g., number of proteges)
   How is your performance measured?_____

d. Employing ethical methods in achieving goals (e.g., complying with ACHE's *Code of Ethics*)

   How is your performance measured?_____

e. Please specify any other criteria regarding professional role fulfill-ment.

_____

5. Are the above criteria subject to modification over the course of the evaluation period?

   Yes...1
   No..2

   Please proceed to question 7.

6. If your performance is NOT evaluated using pre-established written criteria, How is your performance measured?

_____
_____
_____
_____

7. Is your salary and/or bonus tied to your evaluation? (Circle all that apply.)

   Salary...1
   Bonus...2
   Neither..3

8. Please indicate your response by circling one number on each line:

	Strongly disagree	Disagree	Neutral	Agree	Strongly agree
I feel that my current appraisal process is fair	1	2	3	4	5
CEOs should be evaluated by others on the management team	1	2	3	4	5
CEOs should be evaluated by physicians on the hospital's medical staff	1	2	3	4	5
No one can really appreciate what I accomplish for the hospital	1	2	3	4	5

9. Finally, on the lines below, please tell us how you think your current appraisal process could be improved. If you wish us to attribute a quote to you, **please sign your statement**.

_____

_____

_____

_____

_____

_____

_____

_____

_____

Signature: Your signature allows ACHE to use your statement in publications and summaries of this survey

Thank you for completing this survey. Please fax your response to Peter Weil, vice president of Research and Development, ACHE, at (312) 424–0023 by October 24, 2001.

page 4 of 4

CEO Evaluation Forms

**CASE STUDY 2.1: St. John's Lutheran Hospital, Libby, MT
(Reprinted with permission)**

Performance Review Feedback: Rick Palagi, CEO
(Medical Staff, Administrative Team, Department Managers)

Strongly Disagree	Disagree	Neutral	Agree	Strongly Agree
1	2	3	4	5

Does he provide you with the leadership you expect?
Comments:

Does he contribute to the sense of team throughout the hospital?
Comments:

Does he have the respect of hospital staff/people with whom he works?
Comments:

Does he follow through with communications and commitments in a timely fashion?
Comments:

Is he responsive in a timely fashion to your needs, recommendations, etc?
Comments:

Does he have the respect of the Medical Staff?
Comments:

Please list any suggestions for Rick to improve or other comments on any of the above questions.

CEO ANNUAL EVALUATION BOARD OF TRUSTEES FORM

DIRECTIONS – *Below are listed the eight accountability areas on Rick's Position Description. Please place a number in the blank outside each area as to your judgement of his performance using the following scale:*

Strongly Disagree	Disagree	Neutral	Agree	Strongly Agree
1	2	3	4	5

In addition, any comments you have can be added in the comment box. Please return to Karen Stickney in the enclosed envelope by Friday, September 27th.

___ 1. **Strategic Leadership**: Works with the Board, employees and physicians to develop a relevant and compelling written Vision and Mission for the institution. In collaboration with management staff, Board and physician creates and coordinates Strategic Plan and annual Team Action Plans and implements it accordingly, providing regular feedback to the Board on progress being made. Provides proactive, sound guidance to maneuver the institution into the most advantageous position. Evokes respect by Board, peers, medical staff, employees and community. Always seeks win/win solutions. Is persuasive and convincing, is fair and impartial, sets high standards, establishes a clear focus and direction, implements company policies, tackles tough issues. Thinks strategically, possesses vision, has the ability to adjust to change, build advantageous coalitions and foster team spirit in the institution.
Comments:

___ 2. **Quality Improvement and Compliance**: Ensures overall hospital-wide quality and compliance programs are actively in place for all services and facilities. Develops and coordinates systems to monitor and improve clinical quality of care and satisfaction of services rendered. Actively engaged in assuring all legal and regulatory mandates are met. Personally involved with and appropriately delegates patient/family complaints to resolution. Maintains adequate first hand knowledge of patient and family opinions of their care experience.
Comments:

___ 3. **Financial Responsibility**: Displays leadership in financial management from conceptual strategies through recommending policy, executing fiscal procedures for control and effective utilization of physical and financial resources of the hospital. Employs a system of responsible accounting, including budget and internal controls with assistance from the Chief Financial Officer. Creates value by recommending appropriate

actions and strategies to respond to projected economic and utilization trends within the organization.
Comments:

—— 4. **People Management:** Defines roles and responsibilities, motivates and challenges employees, delegates effectively, rewards contributions, manages collaboratively. Regularly schedules and facilitates staff, employee and departmental meetings. Names appropriate departmental representatives to multi-disciplinary committees of the hospital. Applies clear, consistent performance standards, handles performance problems decisively and objectively, is direct but tactful and provides guidance and assistance to improve performance. Establishes formal means of accountability for assigned duties. Promotes a work environment that reflects a positive atmosphere, high employee satisfaction and competence, and strong evidence of teamwork.
Comments:

—— 5. **Board Relations:** Prepares reports for and attends meetings with governing body, realizing the focal point of policy-making is the Board of Directors. Achieves cooperation with the Board by mailing clear cut and precise meeting agendas in advance with appropriate background information and recommendations to Board members. Prepares management recommendations in advance so they can be acted upon by the policy-making body, guarding against "surprises" occurring during the Board meeting, anticipating key questions and achieving a smooth working relationship with the Board Chair.
Comments:

—— 6. **Physician Relations**: Strives to develop an effective, collaborative partnership with the medical staff to maintain communications and positive momentum. Meets routinely with physicians individually and at appropriate committee meetings. Develops an understanding of the physician needs, attitudes, and objectives to blend those with the functions and strategic objectives of the hospital. Seeks input on matters that impact the care processes.
Comments:

—— 7. **Communication:** Establishes and communicates clear expectations. Models open, clear, consistent communication. Demonstrates effective listening.
Comments:

—— 8. **Personal development and professionalism:** Models mission, vision, values. Demonstrates "life-long learning" through professional development, continuing education and promotes same for staff. Is compliant with universal competencies as defined in staff performance standards.
Comments:

CASE STUDY 2.2: Atlantic General Hospital, Berlin, MD
(Reprinted with permission)

Atlantic General Hospital/Health System
President/CEO Performance Goals
October 2002/October 2003

A) <u>Board Governance</u>
- 1. *General:*
  - Maintain open communication with the Board.
  - Provide communication to Board Chair on a timely basis
  - Implement all board approved policies
- 2. *Specific:*
  - With board continue to improve Governance process (minimize duplication, focus on finance, quality, and strategic issues).
  - Continue to provide timely and appropriate board education sessions.
  - Continue to meet with each individual board member.

B) <u>Financial</u>
- 1. *General:*
  - meet overall budget objectives
  - monitor and implement necessary changes to achieve financial goals
- 2. *Specific:*
  - monitor LOS
  - interact with HSCRC related to rate case, work towards improved relationships

C) <u>Strategic</u>
- 1. *General:*
  - Assure that the mission and vision are continually supported in all programs and plans.
- 2. *Specific:*
  - Work with the Planning Committee and Board to update strategic plan objectives focusing on global issues and with the Planning and Medical Executive Committee develop recruitment plans for targeted profesionals and achieve targets.
  - Oversee building projects and land development plans.
  - Provide direction to ambulatory surgery and medical office building development

D) <u>Medical Staff</u>
- 1. *General*
  - Reinforce and communicate importance of collaboration between Administration, Board, and medical staff.
- 2. *Specific:*
  - Implement direct and regular communications with AGHS practitioners/physicians, and their office staff.
  - Evaluate option of physician satisfaction survey tool.

- Evaluate process to improve organizational responses, communication, and marketing to all physician offices and practices.
- Develop plan for formal spin off of billing service for physicians.
- Targeted Recruitment Plan
- Develop/Communicate targeted recruitment plan for 2003 and 2004–2006.

E) Regulatory Compliance

1. General:

- Committment to AGH/AGHS meeting all regulatory requirements.

2. Specific:

- Prepare and operationalize efforts for JCAHO survey in 2003.
- Prepare and operationalize plan for HIPAA compliance.

F) Development/Public Relations

1. General:

- Assure that AGH/HS supports mission and is a positive organization in the community.

2. Specific:

- Provide leadership to all development activities including the Capital Campaign, Annual Appeal, and special events.
- Continue to participate in community civic meeting groups and organizations.
- Expand comunity health/wellness programs.
- Focus marketing plan on approved image criteria.

G) Quality/Safety

1. General:

- Assure that the organization continues to focus on quality and safety as primary.

2. Specific:

- Finalize and implement patient safety plan.
- Continue to refine quality-reporting information to the Board through the Board Quality Assurance Committee.
- Develop organized safety and disaster preparation plan.
- Continue to evaluate expansion of security services.
- Update and finalize patient satisfaction surveys.
- Continue to develop customer service programs.

H) Human Resources

1. General:

- Keep working toward AGH/AGHS as employer of choice.

2. Specific:

- Develop motivational incentive programs for all levels of organization.

CASE STUDY 2.3: Bay Area Medical Center, Marinette, WI
(Reprinted with permission)

CEO Evaluation Guide

CEO Evaluation — Section I
Dimensions/Characteristics of Performance

Using the following definitions of levels of performance, please indicate below your perceptions and evaluations of your CEO's work performance. Mark only those categories in which you feel able to evaluate his/her performance. Additional written comments can be made.

Excellent (E)	Performance is clearly outstanding. Performance is superior—it far exceeds standards or expectations. Performance is exceptional on a continuous basis.
Good (G)	Performance generally meets or exceeds standards or expectations. Attains all or nearly all of position objectives.
Satisfactory (S)	Performance is adequate—it meets standards or expectations and is developing within the position.
Needs Improvement (I)	Fails to meet one or a few job expectations.
Unacceptable (U)	Performance is below accepted levels. Fails to meet most job expectations.
No Basis for Judgment (J)	Have not observed this skill or activity.

1. Leadership and Managerial Qualities	E	G	S	I	U	J
Functions as a self-starter, setting high personal standards and pursuing goals with a high level of personal drive and energy.	E	G	S	I	U	J
Functions as an effective member of a work group, gaining the respect and cooperation of others.	E	G	S	I	U	J
Demonstrates the leadership, initiative, and persistence needed to accomplish goals and objectives.	E	G	S	I	U	J
Assigns tasks to personnel capable of carrying them out.	E	G	S	I	U	J
Establishes clear vision and direction for the organization.	E	G	S	I	U	J
Creates an organizational culture that is needed to carry out the mission, strategic directions and organizational goals.	E	G	S	I	U	J
Monitors current budget and operational data to assure continued success of the organization.	E	G	S	I	U	J
Challenges, motivates, evaluates, and rewards employees and managers toward the achievement of goals and objectives.	E	G	S	I	U	J
Handles problems in a professional manner.	E	G	S	I	U	J

Bay Area continued

2. Knowledge and Skills

Demonstrates thorough knowledge and understanding of hospital management and operations.	E	G	S	I	U	J
Assures that the hospital's quality assurance plan is reviewed and revised as necessary on an annual basis.	E	G	S	I	U	J
Assures the hospital is in accordance with applicable standards, codes, laws, and regulations.	E	G	S	I	U	J
Anticipates trends and opportunities affecting hospital operations and develops an appropriate and timely response.	E	G	S	I	U	J

3. Planning

Develops and maintains a strategic plan for the organization and for the local community.	E	G	S	I	U	J
Develops alternative strategies when current environment changes.	E	G	S	I	U	J
Monitors progress of plan with Board, Medical Staff, and community.	E	G	S	I	U	J

4. Board Relations

Works closely with board of trustees in developing the mission and long- and short-range strategic plans.	E	G	S	I	U	J
Communicates well with the board of trustees, providing appropriate information at and between meetings.	E	G	S	I	U	J
Works with board of trustees to create an optimal governance environment.	E	G	S	I	U	J
Assesses the hospital financial condition, providing complete reports to the board of trustees on a monthly basis.	E	G	S	I	U	J
Supports the policies, procedures, and philosophy of the board of trustees.	E	G	S	I	U	J
Creates a sense of trustworthiness in Board/CEO relations.	E	G	S	I	U	J

5. Medical Staff Relations

Has a good rapport with the medical staff.	E	G	S	I	U	J
Communicates with and works closely with the medical staff members on matters of mutual concern.	E	G	S	I	U	J
Is an effective liaison between the board and medical staff.	E	G	S	I	U	J

6. Community Relations/Political Effectiveness

Develops programs promoting a positive image of hospital, and creates awareness of available services to local community.	E	G	S	I	U	J
Represents the hospital in community activities.	E	G	S	I	U	J
Has the respect of his/her peers in local and state health care organizations.	E	G	S	I	U	J
Maintains an active advocacy role in promoting the needs of the institution and its mission.	E	G	S	I	U	J
Effectively communicates activities of the hospital to the residents of the hospital service area.	E	G	S	I	U	J

Other comments:

Bay Area continued

CEO Evaluation—Section II
Strengths and Development Needs

Based on the responses from Section I:

What are the CEO's major strengths? (List 2 or 3)
1.
2.
3.

What are the areas that need further development? (List 2 or 3)
1.
2.
3.

What assistance or resources are needed to address developmental needs?

CEO Evaluation—Section III
Overall Performance

Excellent   Good   Acceptable   Needs Improvement   Unacceptable

CEO Evaluation—Attachment I
A list of current years goals for the CEO (personal) and hospital (organizational) and the status of accomplishment/completion should be done by the CEO and provided to the trustees prior to the evaluation.
Status of Current Goals for _____
Goal/Status

CEO Evaluation—Attachment II
The board chair/evaluation committee in conjunction with the CEO should list and discuss CEO (personal) and organizational (hospital) goals for the coming year.
Personal and Organizational Goals for _____

CASE STUDY 2.4: Keokuk Health Systems, Keokuk, IA
(Reprinted with permission)

Chief Executive Officer Performance Appraisal Form

Keokuk Health System	2001

Each Director/Trustee is expected to evaluate the performance of the Chief Executive Officer on the following areas of responsibility. Your participation is important to the process and please respond to each area from your own perspective.

1. The CEO directs the organization in a manner consistent with the established Mission Statement.
   ① Poor   ② Fair   ③ Good   ④ Excellent
   Comments:_____

2. The CEO effectively manages the financial resources of the organization to obtain optimal results.
   ① Poor   ② Fair   ③ Good   ④ Excellent
   Comments:_____

3. The CEO manages the organization in compliance with required statutes, regulations, accrediting bodies and in such a manner that minimizes risk of all types to the organization.
   ① Poor   ② Fair   ③ Good   ④ Excellent
   Comments:_____

4. The CEO achieves expected levels of accomplishments on the organization's annual objectives and goals.
   ① Poor   ② Fair   ③ Good   ④ Excellent
   Comments:_____

5. The CEO insures that the organization is staffed with and retains appropriate numbers of motivated, competent professional and support staff members to meet the needs and objectives of the organization.
   ① Poor   ② Fair   ③ Good   ④ Excellent
   Comments:_____

6. The CEO through his management responsibilities assures that the organization's facilities, equipment and physical assets are appropriate, safe and adequate for the services provided.

7. The organization's marketing plans and programs are coordinated, effective and achieve desired results.

① Poor   ② Fair   ③ Good   ④ Excellent

Comments:_____

_____

8. The CEO is an effective communicator with the Governing Board on which I serve.

① Poor   ② Fair   ③ Good   ④ Excellent

Comments:_____

_____

9. The CEO represents the organization with all strategic constituencies and "publics" in an effective manner. i.e. KEDC, Rotary, Chamber, Auxiliary, etc.

① Poor   ② Fair   ③ Good   ④ Excellent

Comments:_____

_____

_____

Each Director/Trustee is asked to provide their input on each of the following issues:

1. This CEO Performance Appraisal Form provides me the opportunity to adequately provide input into the evaluation of the Chief Executive Officer.

① Poor   ② Fair   ③ Good   4 Excellent

Comments:_____

_____

_____

2. From your perspective as a Director/Trustee, what are the three (3) top priorities/objectives to be addressed by this organization in the next year.

#1: _____

#2: _____

#3: _____

Please return this evaluation in the enclosed envelope by <u>Friday, November 16th</u>. Thank you for your participation and input.

Signed:_____

      (Signature optional)

CASE STUDY 2.5: Wadley Regional Medical Center, Texarkana, TX
(Reprinted with permission)

Evaluation of CEO by Board of Directors
2003

	LOW			HIGH	2001	2000	1989–1999
	1	2	3	4	5	Score	Score	Average

1. Understands the role of the medical center in American Society
2. Determines and writes medical center objectives
3. Utilizes board policies to achieve medical center objectives
4. Develops work programs for the medical center
5. Understands the staffing requirements of the medical center
6. Understands the financial requirements of a medical center
7. Generates financial resources for the medical center
8. Allocates medical center resources via the budget
9. Communicates medical center objectives to the staff
10. Anticipates and overcomes barriers to attainment of objectives
11. Delegates authority and responsibility to his staff
12. Releases and focuses capabilities of staff members
13. Maintains communication among staff, board and community
14. Overcomes limitations of staff members
15. Motivates the staff to achieve excellence
16. Makes clear job assignments

	LOW			HIGH		2001	2000	1989–1999
	1	2	3	4	5	Score	Score	Average

17. Solicits suggestions for improved medical center performance
18. Works well with others
19. Likes to solve problems
20. Makes sound decisions
21. Finishes assignments in a timely manner
22. Demonstrates creativity in reaching medical center objectives
23. Monitors medical center performance
24. Recruits capable staff
25. Encourages professional development of employees
26. Anticipates effects of management decisions
27. Insists on high standards
28. Enables the board to work effectively
29. Facilitates effective communication
30. Is always prepared for Board meetings
31. Gives effective verbal presentations
32. Writes effective reports
33. Is sensitive to political issues
34. Maintains necessary correspondence
35. Keeps in touch with the various publics of the medical center
36. Maintains a favorable community image
37. Cooperates with other community groups
38. Promotes medical center interests at national, state and local levels
39. Issues unambiguous and fair decisions
40. Makes impartial decisions

Wadley continued

	LOW				HIGH	2001 Score	2000 Score	1989–1999 Average
	1	2	3	4	5			

41. Follows up on all staff directives
42. Maintains a high level of personal productivity
43. Budgets personal time well
44. Demonstrates punctuality in keeping appointments
45. Provides timely and accurate information in response to inquiries
46. Works well with the medical staff
47. Maintains an aura of easy approachability
48. Follows his/her own admonitions
49. Strives for high quality patient care
50. Strives for medical center cost effectiveness
51. Supervises others effectively
52. Works well with third party agencies
53. Engages in personal and professional development
54. Is liked by most medical center employees
55. Improves personal proficiency through reading and study
56. Makes accurate statements about his/her work
57. Keeps personal problems out of the job
58. Makes a favorable impression upon others
59. Is viewed by the staff and community as a leader
60. Rewards employee performance
61. Maintains professional poise and bearing
62. Sees the "big picture"
63. Presents convincingly a point of view

	LOW				HIGH	2001	2000	1989–1999
	1	2	3	4	5	Score	Score	Average

64. Stays up-to-date on changes affecting medical centers
65. Learns quickly
66. Handles stress
67. Is tolerant of others
68. Is a good business person
69. Is sensitive to other people's feelings
70. Expectations of employees are realistic
71. Works well with the board
72. Is cooperative even under stress
73. Strives for personal excellence
74. Takes criticism well
75. Obviously enjoys the job
76. Is training an understudy
77. Can spot potential legal problems
78. Works well with nursing
79. Maintains an attractive physical plant
80. Is a natural peacemaker
81. Places medical center objectives before personal convenience
82. Is a good fundraiser

CASE STUDY 2.6: Central DuPage Health System, Winfield, IL
(Reprinted with permission)

Evaluation Form
Completed by Board of Directors and Medical Staff

Memorandum

TO: Central DuPage Health System Board of Directors
Central DuPage Hospital Medical Staff Leaders
Central DuPage Health System Executive Team

FROM: Chair
Central DuPage Health Board of Directors

SUBJECT: President and Chief Executive Officer Performance Evaluation

One of our important responsibilities as leaders of Central DuPage Health is to provide a concise and thorough assessment of the performance of Don Sibery in his role as President and Chief Executive Officer. Please participate in the data gathering for this evaluation.

In order for us to get the most valid response possible, I encourage you to use your experience with Don, your recollection of key occurances, and the attached list of "accomplishments" as the substance for making your ratings. I also encourage you to use the response option of "no basis" for rating Don's performance if you feel you do not have sufficient knowledge for formulating a rating.

An evaluation form comparable to this one will be used by physician leaders, members of the Central DuPage Health Board of Directors, and members of the System Executive Team (SET). Please verify that you have received an evaluation form that accurately reflects the group you are part of. In the case of dual designations, we will give you the questionnaire that matches your primary function.

Because we appreciate any comments you have, we have allocated space for you to write your remarks. I hope you will feel free to contact me if you would like to discuss your comments. Only overall results will be shared with Don. Your individual evaluation will remain confidential.

I want to thank you in advance for your time and input.

The overall performance rating scheme is described on the following page.

I. Introduction and Instructions

For each of the key responsibilities listed below, please identify the rating that best indicates the way you feel about the effectiveness of the President and CEO's performance. If you believe you have no basis for evaluation leave the response blank. Please feel free to comment in the space provided after each area of responsibility, and at the end of this evaluation, particularly if you believe there are areas for which improvement in performance is required. At the end of each responsiblity area (e.g., Management/Employee Relations), you may give an overall rating. Please note this is not a simple average of the sub-area rating for that area, rather it is your rating of your overall impression of Don Sibery's performance in the area of responsibility.

Please return your completed evaluation form to me in the confidential envelope provided no later than May 18, 2001.

Your information will be compiled with that received from other key stakeholders and will be used by the Board's Executive Committee in completing the overall performance evaluation for the President and CEO.

Performance Rating	Definition
Exceeds Expectations	Performance is clearly above the norm and consistently exceeds the expected performance level of the standard or objective.
Meets Expectations	Performance meets level of expectations of the standard or objective. Performance is fully satisfactory.
Requires Improvement	Performance is marginally acceptable and is inconsistent in meeting the expectations of the health system in this standard or objective. Please comment on the specific reason(s) for your evaluation.
No Basis	No experience or knowledge for assigning a value.

II. Key Responsibilities

	Exceeds Expectations	Meets Expectations	Requires Improvement	No Basis
A. BOARD OF DIRECTORS RELATIONS				
1. Involves the Board in the strategic planning process.				
2. Provides the Board of Directors with assessments of changes in the business environment affecting the strategic plan.				
3. Keeps the Board apprised of important operational, legal, and governmental issues as they relate to oversight of the health care system				

	Exceeds Expect- ations	Meets Expect- ations	Requires Improve- ment	No Basis

4   Encourages the continuting education and development of each Board member.

5. Coordinates the continuing education and development of each Board member.

6. Ensures that a process is in place for ongoing review of the performance of the Board.

7. Ensures that a process is in place for ongoing review of the performance of individual Board members.

8. Ensures that the Board and its Committees are provided with sufficient background material supplied in a timely fashion so that the Board is able to carry out its fiduciary duties.

9. Annually provides the board the opportunity for a thorough orientation to Board policies and procedures, and an overview of Central DuPage Health's operations.

10. Maintains a productive working relationship with members of the Board of Directors.

11. Provides appropriate follow-up reports to the Board outlining the progress made in implementing these plans.

12. Overall impression of the President and CEO's performance in the area of Board relations.

Comments:

B. PHYSICIAN RELATIONS

1. Ensures a plan is in place for physician development.

2. Encourages physician leadership throughout the health care system.

3. Maintains effective communications with the physician leadership in the medical community.

4. Maintains a productive working relationship with the physician leadership.

	Exceeds Expect- ations	Meets Expect- ations	Requires Improve- ment	No Basis

5. Involves key members of the medical community in the strategic planning process for the health care system.
6. Works effectively with the leadership of physician organizations in the health care system's market area.
7. Encourages input from physicians; e.g., key operational issues and strategic plans.
8. Develops physician leaders through their membership on task forces, formal education, and continuing education.
9. Overall impression of the President and CEO's performance in the area of physician relations.

Comments:

C. MANAGEMENT/EMPLOYEE RELATIONS

1. Recruits, develops, and encourages retention of executive management.
2. Ensures that executive management works effectively with each other, the Board of Directors, and the medical community.
3. Ensures selection and employment practices which hold people accountable.
4. Empowers staff to lead.
5. Fosters an environment of quality service.
6. Fosters an environment of acknowledgment.
7. Fosters an environment of listening.
8. Fosters an environment of partnership and teamwork.
9. Anticipates Central DuPage Health's work force needs for the future.
10. Overall impression of the President and CEO's performance in the area of management/employee relations.

Comments:

	Exceeds Expect- ations	Meets Expect- ations	Requires Improve- ment	No Basis

D. COMMUNITY, ORGANIZATION, AND GOVERNMENT RELATIONS

1. Establishes and maintains effective relationships with local, regional, state, and federal organizations and officials which influence the health care system's ability to serve its community.
2. Ensures the health care system is a world class "corporate citizen."
3. Ensures the organization meets its obligations as a major employer in the area to provide human and other resources in support of community initiatives (e.g., United Way, Chambers of Commerce, community task forces, Boards of Directors of various non-profit organizations, etc.)
4. Overall impression of the President and CEO's performance in the area of community, organization, and government relations.

Comments:

E. SYSTEM MEMBER ORGANIZATIONS' BOARDS OF DIRECTORS RELATIONS

1. Communicates effectively the health care system's strategy and its impact upon member organizations.
2. Participates in Board meetings in such a way that he supports the member organizations' leadership.
3. Encourages "systemness" in decision making.
4. Represents fairly, accurately, and in a timely fashion the needs and requests of member organization Boards directed to system leadership and the system Board.
5. Overall impression of the President and CEO's performance in the area of system member organizations' Boards of Directors relations.

	Exceeds Expect- ations	Meets Expect- ations	Requires Improve- ment	No Basis

Comments:

F. QUALITY OF CARE AND SERVICE
The President and CEO ensures that:
1. the resources of the health care system are organized and managed in such a manner that quality is measurable;
2. Central DuPage Health's outcomes are compared against acceptable benchmarks;
3. Central DuPage Health is continually improving the processes of care and service;
4. the continuum of care is enhanced;
5. the community's health is measurably being optimized;
6. the appropriate parties work to accomplish successful accreditation, licensure, and certification by relevant outside reviewing bodies; and,
7. the customer's needs and expectations of the health care system are met.
8. Overall impression of the President and CEO's performance in the area of quality of care and service.
Comments:

G. PLANNING
He ensures that plans, goals, and objectives exist for the following:
1. business strategy;
2. equipment and facilities;
3. information technology;
4. human resources; and,
5. capital requirements.
6. The President and CEO includes key stakeholders in developing these plans.
7. Overall impression of the President and CEO's performance in the area of planning.
Comments:

	Exceeds Expect- ations	Meets Expect- ations	Requires Improve- ment	No Basis

H. FINANCIAL STEWARDSHIP

The President and CEO ensures that:

1. the five-year capital requirements plan spells out essential assumptions regarding operating costs, capital equipment, facilities, information technology, community health initiatives, working capital, volumes, pricing, and profitability.

2. financial operations are carried out in a manner which supports the health care system's mission and strategic plan;

3. an effective operating and capital budget process for the health care system is in place;

4. the health care system's operations are carried out within the intent of the budget;

5. appropriate, comparative financial benchmarks are utilized thereby enabling the management and the Board to assess the overall financial health of the health care system in comparison to the external benchmarks;

6. through the scope and quality of the audit function the community's assets are being safeguarded;

7. assets are deployed consistent with the health care system's non-profit status and mission; and

8. managed care contracting policies and procedures are contemporary (e.g., they align incentives among providers, they encourage innovation and appropriate use of resources, they allow for appropriate risk-taking, and they reward parties for their efforts).

9. Overall impression of the President and CEO's performance in the area of financial stewardship.

Comments:

I. OPERATIONS

1. The President and CEO ensures the health care system's operations are

Central DuPage continued

	Exceeds Expect- ations	Meets Expect- ations	Requires Improve- ment	No Basis

carried out in a manner which supports the objectives and mission of the system.

2. He ensures that the health care system's facilities and campuses present a positive, clean, and professional appearance.

3. He also ensures that the health care system's operations demonstrate attention to quality and courteous service.

4. The President and CEO is fully engaged in the implementation of the Centered Around You philosophy in the health care system's operations.

5. Overall impression of the President and CEO's performance in the area of operations.

Comments

III. Summary Comments

_____
_____
_____
_____
_____
_____
_____
_____

Name (optional)

Author's Note: The evaluation form completed by the medical staff leaders excludes items A and E above.

CASE STUDY 2.7: Overlake Hospital Medical Center, Bellevue, WA   (Reprinted with permission)

CEO Performance Review "Key Stakeholder" Input Form
August 2002

Key: A = "Above and Beyond" (value added) contributor in this area
B = Fully competent contributor in this area
C = Cannot rate
D = Does not contribute fully in this area

Area of Evaluation   **A   B   C   D**

Board Relations. Keeps the OHA Board well informed. No surprises. Assists the COO in relations with the OHMC Board as needed. Seeks input from the Board(s) as appropriate. Follows through on items assigned by Board(s). Helps the Board with decision making and problem solving as appropriate.

Medical Staff/Physician Relations. Communicates effectively with physicians. Is available to medical staff as may be needed. Maintains the respect of the medical staff.

Employee Relations. Sets the tone for an OHA culture which attracts and retains well performing employees. Insures that all employees are treated with respect, honesty, and integrity. Is recognized as an effective leader by employees. Instills an organization-wide sense of "team."

Advocacy for Quality and Mission. Maintains a focus on mission while pursuing financial/market success. Requires the organization to objectively measure quality levels. Continually encourages improvement in service levels.

Articulating Organization Direction. Creates a vision of the future for the overall organization. Enrolls the board, Physicians, and staff in support of the vision. Establishes goals and action plans to "operationalize" the vision.

Innovation and Flexibility. Insures that the organization pursues new programs and services to meet market needs. Responds to issues and problems with adaptive, creative solutions/responses. A leader in responding positively to change, and helping others to do so.

Leadership of OHA Executive Team. Demonstrates team building and conflict resolution skills with executives. Selects and develops executives successfully. Maintains a results-oriented culture with the executive team, including performance management.

Area of Evaluation   **A   B   C   D**

Leadership in External Relations. Establishes/maintains effective relations with the community. Establishes/maintains effective relations with government and regulatory agencies. Encourages and pursues long-term affiliations which fit into OHA's strategic plans.

Fiscal Responsibility. Achieves financial goals as set by the Board. Promotes effective allocation and utilization of resources. Insures the development of long-term financial plans for the organization.

Operational Leadership. Insures that others put appropriate monitoring, measurement, and corrective action systems in place. Takes corrective action when needed. Is knowledgeable about key operating issues, while maintaining a primary focus on strategic leadership.

Fund Raising. Works effectively with the Foundation Executive Director and Foundation Board. Maintains positive relations with major donors. Provides meaningful support to major fundraising activities.

Comments:

Performance Review, Employee Performance Review and Development Plan for Hospital-based Associates

Employee Name   Hospital & Location

Position Title   Group Vice President/Division

Purpose: **Annual Evaluation**   **Other**

Directions: This form is to be used to evaluate the performance of hospital-based employees. The supervisor should evaluate only those performance areas observed.

Supervisor's Signature   Date

Group VP or Division SVP's Signature   Date

This performance review and development plan has been discussed with me.

Employee's Signature   Date

ACHIEVEMENT OF ESTABLISHED OBJECTIVES/RESPONSIBILITIES:
Summarize the overall effectiveness in meeting position objectives and fulfilling ongoing position responsibilities. Comments should include *specific examples* of accomplished and/or not accomplished objectives/responsibilities.

MANAGEMENT RESULTS: (for supervisory review): Record major performance results achieved in the supervision of others, include such items as staffing, delegating, motivating, resulting conflict, developing subordinates, etc. *Comments and Specific Examples:

Northwestern Medical continued

ETHICS AND COMPLIANCE: Summarize activity which demonstrates that the employee meets the required annual Compliance Training standard specific to his or her job. Comment on how the employee adheres to the Quorum Health Resources Code of Conduct.

COMMENTS ON RESULTS: The way an employee works to achieve results can often positively or negatively affect his/her performance or the performance of others. Comment on the methods and approach used by the employee in performing his/her job.

Employee performance is often beneficially or adversely influenced by conditions beyond their control. Comments on any circumstances which should be considered in reviewing employee performance results for this period. How did employee handle these conditions?

OVERALL PERFORMANCE RATING:

_____ Outstanding
_____ Exceeds
_____ Satisfactory
_____ Below

COMPETENCY PROFILE

Competency Rating: Use the following scale to rate the employee on the profile criteria indicated below. For each profile criteria, choose the rating that best represents the typical effectiveness of this employee in his/her position.

5 Extremely Effective
4 Very Effective
3 Effective
2 Somewhat Effective
1 Not Effective
0 Not Applicable

Functional

1. Operations _____
2. Marketing _____
3. Finance _____
4. Data Processing _____
5. Technical _____
6. Labor Relations _____
7. Community Relations _____
8. Government Relations _____
9. Physician Relations _____
10. Corporate Relations _____
11. Board Relations _____
12. International _____
13. _____ _____
14. _____ _____
15. _____ _____
16. _____ _____

Managerial

17. Strategy _____
18. Planning/Organizing _____
19. Control _____
20. Staff mgmt/Development _____
21. Policy _____

Environmental

22. External Relations _____
23. Economics _____
24. Customer Awareness _____

Leadership

25. Corporate Culture _____
26. Leadership Styles _____
27. Compliance & Code of Conduct _____

Interpersonal

28. Oral Communication _____
29. Written Communications _____
30. Political Awareness _____
31. Negotiating _____
32. Health Management _____
33. Stress Management _____

Decision Making

34. Analytical Approaches _____
35. Decision Methods _____
36. Judgement/Decisiveness _____
37. Social Contributions _____
38. Entrepreneurship _____
39. Creativity _____

Comments by Supervisor: Describe and cite examples where the employee has demonstrated superior behavior, abilities, knowledge, interest, etc. Likewise, comment on any improvements expected in specific competencies.

Development Plan

Recommended Future Position(s) based upon Performance: List position(s) in priority order:

Type of Position	Hospital or Corporate	Location	Timing
1			
2			

Recommended Development Activities: List up to two job activities that would be beneficial to the employee's development in the coming year (e.g., non-classroom activities such as serving on task forces, boards, committees, etc.) Give dates for developing activity.

Development Activity (on-the-job)	Start Date	End Date
1		
2		

Northwestern Medical continued

List up to two formal classroom activities that would be beneficial to the employee's development (e.g., university courses, seminars, programs, etc.) Give date each activity is scheduled to start.

Educational Activity (Classroom)	Start Date	End Date
1		
2		

Comments by Supervisor: Comment on recommended next position(s) and development activities. Provide explanation in situations where there are no recommendations (e.g., appropriately placed, not available for transfer, etc.)

To be completed by employee
Individual Preferences: List your own preferences regarding future positions.

Type of Position	Hospital or Corporate	Location	Timing
1			
2			

Willingness to relocate: (check one)

_____ Limited _____ Unlimited _____ Will not relocated at this time

Comments by employee: Comment on your preferences for future positions and/or your mobility.

COMMENTS BY THE EMPLOYEE: Give overall comments on your review.

Northwestern Medical continued

POSITION OBJECTIVES FORM

Date of Review: _____   Name of Associate: _____

Position Held: _____   Hospital/Location: _____

Objectives	Performance Standards/Measures	Results Achieved (Including explanation of variances)
No. 1		
No. 2		
No. 3		

Northwestern Medical continued

Objectives	Performance Standards/Measures	Results Achieved (Including explanation of variances)
No. 4		
No. 5		
No. 6		
No. 7		

CASE STUDY 3.2: MountainView Hospital, Las Vegas, NV
(Reprinted with permission)

**MountainView Hospital
Board of Trustees**

Evaluation of the Chief Executive Officer

2001

The attached statements and questions are designed to evaluate the performance of the Chief Executive Officer during the past year and to elicit your response to his performance. Inclusion of your name is **Optional**, however it would be helpful to indicate the number of months/years you have served as a Trustee.

Ratings will start with a number 1 for **Strongly Agree** and will diminish to a number 4 for **Disagree**; the **NS** will indicate that you are **Not Sure**. The **Ratings** for each section will be averaged to determine a high and low score. Please remember that your answer should only reflect Board activity for the past year. You are encouraged to comment on any or all of the questions.

I = **Strongly Agree**   4 = **Disagree**   NS = **Not Sure**

Section I: Board Relations

I   2   3   4   NS

☐   ☐   ☐   ☐   ☐   A. Is there a yearly review of the hospital mission statement with the Board?

☐   ☐   ☐   ☐   ☐   B. Is timely information provided to the Board?

☐   ☐   ☐   ☐   ☐   C. Is Board policy successfully implemented?

☐   ☐   ☐   ☐   ☐   D. Is Board planning facilitated through education and timely communication?

☐   ☐   ☐   ☐   ☐   E. Is the Board kept informed in regards to hospital operations?

Section II: Finance

I   2   3   4   NS

☐   ☐   ☐   ☐   ☐   A. Was an acceptable budget prepared and presented to the Board for approval on time?

☐   ☐   ☐   ☐   ☐   B. Did the hospital's financial outcome meet or exceed approved budget targets for the prior fiscal year?

☐   ☐   ☐   ☐   ☐   C. Is the hospital meeting the long-term objectives for new and improved services and programs and realizing the projected financial benefits from these objectives?

☐   ☐   ☐   ☐   ☐   D. Are costs being contained relative to productivity, volume and quality of care?

Section III: Planning

I   2   3   4   NS

☐   ☐   ☐   ☐   ☐   A. Has an effective short-term and long-range institutional plan been developed and communicated to the Board?

☐   ☐   ☐   ☐   ☐   B. Has the planning process served the hospital well for purposes of positioning itself in the community?

☐   ☐   ☐   ☐   ☐   C. Does the planning process serve the hospital well for positioning itself in the community?

☐   ☐   ☐   ☐   ☐   D. Have the Medical Staff and Nursing Staff been effectively integrated into the planning process?

1 = **Strongly Agree**   4 = **Disagree**   NS = **Not Sure**

Section IV: Public–Community Relations/Communications

1	2	3	4	NS	
☐	☐	☐	☐	☐	A. Has the hospital's services been effectively communicated to the community?
☐	☐	☐	☐	☐	B. Are the hospital's needs effectively communicated to the internal organization (medical and nursing staffs, other personnel, Board, volunteers)?
☐	☐	☐	☐	☐	C. Are the hospital's needs represented in the Legislature?
☐	☐	☐	☐	☐	D. Is Board policy successfully implemented?
☐	☐	☐	☐	☐	E. Have there been appropriate efforts made to educate the public on health awareness (diabetes, CPR, etc.)?

Section V: Medical Staff Relations

1	2	3	4	NS	
☐	☐	☐	☐	☐	A. Maintains an organized relationship with the Medical Staff for clinical leadership and compliance with JCAHO, state and federal policy and regulation.
☐	☐	☐	☐	☐	B. Promotes teamwork among the Medical Staff and hospital.
☐	☐	☐	☐	☐	C. Maintains community physician needs through physician recruitment.
☐	☐	☐	☐	☐	D. Fosters physician trust and confidentiality.

Section VI: Management

1	2	3	4	NS	
☐	☐	☐	☐	☐	A. Meets and directs administrative management and middle management.
☐	☐	☐	☐	☐	B. Develops and maintains human resources management.
☐	☐	☐	☐	☐	C. Purchases all appropriate supplies for the operation of the hospital and affiliates.
☐	☐	☐	☐	☐	D. Maintains personal professional status.

1 = **Strongly Agree**   4 = **Disagree**   NS = **Not Sure**

Section VII: Quality/Regulatory Compliance

1	2	3	4	NS	
☐	☐	☐	☐	☐	A. Creates and monitors action systems to continuously and systematically improve compliance with regulatory requirements as set forth by the State of Nevada, federal government and other regulatory agencies.
☐	☐	☐	☐	☐	B. Responds to the hospital's performance improvement program with meaningful action taken toward identified quality issues.
☐	☐	☐	☐	☐	C. Develops and implements strategic plan for continuum of quality patient care.
☐	☐	☐	☐	☐	D. Responds both to patient safety initiatives and care of the environment plans.

Additional Comments

_____

_____

_____

_____

_____

_____

Name (Optional)

_____   _____
Board of Trustee   Date
MountainView Hospital

HCA

PERFORMANCE REVIEW INSTRUCTIONS
Hospital Management Employees

The Performance Review is designed to promote dialogue between employees and supervisors through the use of specific examples. As a performance summary and development tool, it is not intended to be used as initial documentation of performance problems.

PROCESS

The Performance Review form and Performance Review meeting may be completed one of two ways. Choose the most appropriate approach for your situation.

Option A:
1. The supervisor completes the Goals/Objectives part of Section 1.
2. The supervisor provides the employee with a copy of the Performance Review form (with the Goals/Objectives completed) and asks the employee to complete the results assessment (right side of section I), Section III and Section IV.
3. At the same time the supervisor also completes a draft of the results assessment (right side of Secion I), Section II, and Section IV.
4. When the employee submits their assessment, the supervisor compares the employee's assessment to his/her own, analyzes any gaps or disconnects between the two, then composes the final draft, and obtains the department head's signature.
5. The supervisor and the employee will discuss the final assessment at the performance review meeting at which time the employee will sign the final draft. The supervisor and employee should keep copies for their records and submit the orginal to HR.
6. In a later meeting the supervisor and the employee will meet and jointly complete the Goals/Objectives and Development Plan for the coming review period. See *Goals/Objectives and Development Plan* instructions for details.

Option B:
1. The supervisor completes both the Goals/Objectives and the assessment of results in Section I as well as Sections II and IV.

---

2. The supervisor conducts the Performance Review meeting and the employee is given the opportunity to discuss anything with which they do not agree. At that time the employee is asked to take the Performance Review form and provide written comments regarding anything with which they do not agree as well as completing Section III.

3. Once the employee returns their comments, the supervisor composes the final draft. The final draft is signed by all the appropriate persons and is submitted to Human Resources. The supervisor and employee should keep a copy for their records.

4. In a later meeting the supervisor and the employee will meet and jointly complete the Goals/Objectives and Development Plan for the coming review period. See *Goals/Objectives and Development Plan* instructions for details.

FORM COMPLETION

I. **Achievement of Goals/Objectives**—Typically five to six goals/objectives should have been identified by the supervisor and reviewed by the employee at the beginning of the performance period. (See Goals/Objectives and Development Plan instructions for instructions for setting these objectives.) These should be transferred to the left column of section I by the supervisor. The right column in section I should reflect the results the employee achieved (or did not achieve). The final draft should be completed by the supervisor with input from the employee.

II. **Overall Performance Comments**—This section should be completed by the supervisor. It should be a brief narrative describing the employees overall performance.

III. **Employee Comments**—This section should be completed by the employee. It should be a brief narrative describing the employee's perspective regarding his/her overall performance.

IV. **Competency Assessment**—This section is an assessment of how well the employee does or does not demonstrate the desired competencies in the performance of his/her job. Specific examples should be provided, both positive and negative as applicable. A rating should also be assigned using the scale described on the form. *The ECO Competencies field should be completed for all Facility ECO's.*

V. **Signatures**—The reviewer and department head's signatures indicate that they agree with the contents of the appraisal. The employee's signature indicates that the performance appraisal was reviewed with him/her. It does not necessarily indicate that the employee agrees with the contents of the appraisal.

PERFORMANCE REVIEW
Hospital Management Employees

Employee Name and Social Security Number	Location Department
Present Position	Review Period

I. ACHIEVEMENT OF GOALS/OBJECTIVES

The reviewer should list, on the left, the goals/objectives of this position that were identified at the beginning of the review period. These goals/objectives may include basic job responsibilities and/or special projects. The right side of this section should be completed by the reviewer, with input from the employee, to indicate how well each objective was accomplished.

Goals/Objectives	Results/Achievements
1.	1.
2.	2.
3.	3.
4.	4.
5.	5.

II. OVERALL PERFORMANCE COMMENTS

The reviewer should provide a brief assessment of the employee's overall performance.

III. Employee Comments

The employee should provide his/her perspective regarding their performance during the evaluation period.

IV. COMPETENCY ASSESSMENT

The Reviewer should provide examples of how each competency is or is not demonstrated by the employee in the performance of his/her job. Also a space is provided for a rating of the employee's overall effectiveness in each competency area. Each Competency has several definitions which help explain it. It is not necessary to address each definition during the review. It is possible some may not be applicable for this review. This section should be completed by the supervisor with input from the employee. Refer to the HR Public Folder (OUTLOOK) for complete competency definitions. The following ratings should be used:

E=Exceeds Expectations	Exceeds expectations on most objectives; is recognized outside the department as exceptional.
M=Meets Expectations	Meets all objectives; exceeds some; is recognized as a solid performer.
D=Does Not Meet Expectations	Does not meet basic expectations for the job; may still be on the learning curve.
N/A=Not Applicable	This competency does not apply to the incumbent's current job.

Competency	Result(s)	Rating
Integrity: behaves ethically and honestly; supports workplace diversity; communications openly in all directions; balances work life issues; fosters trust in relationships; allocates resources effectively and ethically; actions always consistent with code of conduct. Supports the Ethics and Compliance Program.		
Teamwork: promotes cooperation; builds bridges of cooperation; actively contributes to group efforts; supports team decisions; puts aside self interest; works with diversity.		
Customer & Quality Focus: knows customers and adds value; actively listens; treats customers like business partners; monitors quality and customer satisfaction; delivers to high standards; manages customer expectations.		

Competency	Result(s)	Rating
Development: advocates a learning environment; empowers others; provides frequent and candid feedback; coaches and supports others; fosters an innovative environment.		
Leadership: sets a living example; develops and communicates a shared vision; demonstrates credibility; acts with strategic focus; makes effective decisions; delegates appropriately; selects the right people; thinks beyond today's practice. *ECO's: Encourages a climate of ethical sensitivity and compliant activity.*		
Business Sense: exhibits a health care savvy; gets things done; aligns decisions with values; solves problems; demonstrates professional/ technical knowledge; anticipates challenges and takes risks.		
ECO Competencies: incorporates the values of the Ethics & Compliance Program in the basic cultural fabric of the facility; distributes Code of Conduct and new policies and procedures, and conducts related training; conducts investigations of compliance-related matters; involved in appropriate monitoring and auditing activities; identifies trends which might indicate potential ethics and compliance issues and appropriate actions; conducts regular, effective Facility Ethics and Compliance Committee meetings.		

V. SIGNATURES

Reviewer's Signature	Date	Department Head (prior to employee review)	Date
Signature of employee indicates that the performance appraisal was reviewed with him/her; it does not necessarily indicate that employee agrees with appraisal. ➡		Employee Signature	Date

CASE STUDY 4.1: Yuma District Hospital, Yuma, CO
(Reprinted with permission)

Position Description/Performance Evaluation

Job Title: Chief Executive Officer,   Supervised By: Board of Directors
Acute Care Hospital
Prepared By:_____   Approved By:_____
Date:_____   Date:_____

Job Summary: Manages and directs the organization toward its primary objectives. Establishes current and long range objectives, plans and policies, subject to the approval by the Governing Body. Dispenses advice, guidance, direction and authorization to carry out major plans and procedures, consistent with established policies and Board approval. Oversees the adequacy and soundness of the organization's financial structure. Reviews operating results of the organization, compares them to established objectives, and takes steps to ensure that appropriate measures are taken to correct unsatisfactory results. Represents the organization with major customers, shareholders, the financial community, and the public.

Duties and Responsibilities:
E=Exceeds the Standard   M-Meets the Standard   NI=Needs Improvement

<u>Demonstrates Competency in the Following Areas:</u>	<u>E</u>	<u>M</u>	<u>NI</u>
Responsible for all aspects of the operation of the hospital.	2	1	0
Implements all policies established by the Governing Body; advises during the formation of such policies and reports on the implementation of such policies to the Board.	2	1	0
Develops and submits to the Board for approval a plan of organization for the conduct of the hospital and recommended changes when necessary.	2	1	0
Causes an annual budget to be prepared showing the expected revenue and expenditures as required by the Board.	2	1	0
Selects, employs, controls, and discharges personnel and develops and maintains personnel policies and practices for the hospital.	2	1	0
Ensures maintenance of physical properties in good and safe state of repair and operation.	2	1	0
Supervises the business affairs of the hospital to ensure that funds are collected and expended to the best possible advantage.	2	1	0
Presents to the Board, and/or its committees, periodic reports reflecting the services and financial activities of the hospital and such special reports as may be required by the Board.	2	1	0
Attends all meetings of the Board and its committees, Governing Body.	2	1	0

	E	M	NI

Ensures that the hospital maintains accreditation, licensing and quality patient care through the establishment of performance improvement monitoring programs and standards.   2   1   0

Prepares a plan for the achievement of the hospital's specific objectives and mutually established goals and periodically reviews and evaluates such plan. Said plan shall at all times reflect the hospital's mission statement and be in accordance with the ethics and goals of the hospital.   2   1   0

Act as a liason between the hospital and the medical staff and represents the hospital at external functions.   2   1   0

Performs other duties that may be necessary or in the best interest of the hospital.   2   1   0

Professional Requirements:

Adheres to dress code, appearance is neat and clean.   2   1   0

Completes annual education requirements.

Maintains regulatory requirements, including all state, federal and JCAHO regulations.   2   1   0

Maintains and ensures patient confidentiality at all times.   2   1   0

Reports to work on time and as scheduled.   2   1   0

Wears identification while on duty.   2   1   0

Attends annual review and performs departmental inservices.   2   1   0

Works at maintaining a good rapport and a cooperative working relationship with physicians, departments and staff.   2   1   0

Represents the organization in a positive and professional manner.   2   1   0

Attends committees, CQI and management meetings, as appropriate.   2   1   0

Resolves personnel concerns at the departmental level, utilizing the grievance process as required.   2   1   0

Ensures compliance with policies and procedures regarding deparment operations, fire, safety and infection control.   2   1   0

Effectively and consistently communicates administrative directive to personnel and encourages interactive departmental meetings and discussions.   2   1   0

Complies with all organizational policies regarding ethical business practices.   2   1   0

Communicates the mission, ethics and goals of the facility, as well as the focus statement of the departments.   2   1   0

Total Points   __ __ __

Annual Competency Skills Assessment
Evaluation of Performance
Chief Executive Officer

1=Cannot Perform Skills Independently
2=Requires Some Assistance to Perform Skills
3=Can Perform Skills Independently
NA=Not Applicable

- What procedures have you implemented to promote communication and to enhance the flow of information?   1   2   3   NA

- What procedures do you follow to evaluate overall operations of the facility?   1   2   3   NA

- What protocol is followed when preparing the annual budget, including revenue and expenditures?   1   2   3   NA

- What is your role in an emergency/disaster situation?   1   2   3   NA

- What procedures are followed when reviewing operating results of the organization and correcting unsatisfactory results?   1   2   3   NA

- What are the corporate goals and growth objectives of the facility?   1   2   3   NA

- Implements programs to improve community access to care.   1   2   3   NA

- Demonstrates the ability to plan and direct negotiations pertaining to mergers, joint ventures, acquisition of businesses or the sale of major assets with the approval of the Governing Body.   1   2   3   NA

- Demonstrates the ability to establish long term goals for the facility.   1   2   3   NA

- Expresses a thorough knowledge of all operations of the facility.   1   2   3   NA

- Demonstrates excellent business management.   1   2   3   NA

- Demonstrates a strong working relationship with the COO, medical staff, employees, public groups and the Governing Body.   1   2   3   NA

- Demonstrates/provides thorough knowledge of local, state, federal regulations and JCAHO standards.   1   2   3   NA

- Demonstrates the ability to develop and revise operational policies.   1   2   3   NA

- Demonstrates a commitment to performance improvement and CQI activities.   1   2   3   NA

- Demonstrates strong communication/presentation skills. 1 2 3 NA

- Maintains professional growth and development 1 2 3 NA
  through seminars, workshops and professional
  affiliations.

- Attends and serves on professional/civic service 1 2 3 NA
  organizations as facility representative.

- Facility Environment—Able to locate and/or demonstrate knowledge of:
  - Hospital Departments 1 2 3 NA
  - Hospital Directory 1 2 3 NA
  - Physician Directory 1 2 3 NA
  - Hospital Disaster Plan 1 2 3 NA
  - Fire Equipment:
    - Alarms 1 2 3 NA
    - Extinguishers 1 2 3 NA
    - Exit doors 1 2 3 NA

- Facility Organization—Able to describe roles and functions of:
  - Chief Operating Officer 1 2 3 NA
  - Controller 1 2 3 NA
  - Chief Financial Officer 1 2 3 NA
  - Nursing Executive 1 2 3 NA
  - Governing Body 1 2 3 NA
  - Department Managers 1 2 3 NA
  - Other Departments 1 2 3 NA

- Department(s) Direction:
  - Oversight of management, staff 1 2 3 NA
  - Purchase of physical properties, maintenance 1 2 3 NA
  - Establishes and implements policies 1 2 3 NA
  - Oversees organization's financial structure 1 2 3 NA

- Facility Resources—Locates and demonstrates use of:
  - Reviews and revises Hospital Policy and 1 2 3 NA
    Procedure Manual
  - Administrative Policy and Procedure Manual 1 2 3 NA
  - Fire/Emergency Preparedness Manual 1 2 3 NA
  - Material Safety Data Sheets (MSDS) Manual 1 2 3 NA
  - Safety Manual 1 2 3 NA
  - Individual Department Manuals 1 2 3 NA
  - Specific Reference Materials/Community 1 2 3 NA
    Resources
  - PI Documentation 1 2 3 NA
  - Other 1 2 3 NA

- Facility Routines—Able to demonstrate/provide knowledge of:
  - Communication System:
  - Meetings/Meeting Minutes 1 2 3 NA
  - Memos 1 2 3 NA
  - Reports 1 2 3 NA
  - Represents the organization to the public, 1 2 3 NA
    shareholders, customers and financial
    community.

- Cultural Factors:
  - Religion   1   2   3   NA
  - Food Preferences   1   2   3   NA
  - Family/Community Relationships   1   2   3   NA
  - Healthcare Attitudes/Understanding   1   2   3   NA
  - Trust/Privacy Needs   1   2   3   NA
  - Socioeconomic Environment   1   2   3   NA

Total of Score #3s:_____
Total of Score #2s:_____
Total of Score #1s :_____

Identified Areas that Require Improvement:

_____

_____

_____

_____

_____

_____

Comments:

_____

_____

_____

_____

_____

_____

_____

_____

_____

_____

Name:_____   Title: _____

Date: _____

Signature of Supervisor: _____

Signature of Staff Member: _____

**Performance Evaluation
Continuation Page**

Staff Member: _____ Job Title:_____

Performance Evaluation Score:
# of total points achieved

80–100% exceeds standards
50–79% meets standards

_____ x 100 = _____%

0–49% needs improvement

(# questions x 2)

Manager's Comments:

_____
_____
_____
_____
_____

Recommended Goals/Actions:

_____
_____
_____
_____

Staff Member Comments:

_____
_____
_____

Actions Recommended by Department Manager:
☐ Performance Review Only   ☐ Probation Completed Satisfactorily
☐ Extended Probation Until _____   ☐ Salary Increase Denied
☐ Salary Increase _____

_____   _____
Staff Member Signature   Date

_____   _____
Department Manager Signature   Date

_____   _____
Administrative Signature   Date

Executive Career Field (ECF)
Performance Plan for FY 2003
Network Directors

Introduction

The 2003 Executive Career Field (ECF) Performance Plans consist of Part A
sections 1 and 2, and B. Part A section 1, describes key executive core
competencies, Part A section 2, highlights additional core competencies, and
Part B defines performance measures.

Evaluation of Part A:

Section 1: Key Core Competencies (30 Percent)

The key core competencies are defined as interpersonal effectiveness,
systems thinking, flexibility/adaptability, and organizational stewardship.
At the end of the rating period, Directors will be asked to briefly describe a
personal action/accomplishment that reflects each of these competencies.

Section 2: Core Competencies (20 Percent)

The additional core competencies are defined as creative thinking,
customer service, personal mastery, and technical competency. At the end
of the rating period, Directors will be asked to briefly describe a personal
action/accomplishment that reflects each of these competencies.

Evaluation of Part B: Performance Measures (50 Percent)

The performance measures are categorized by the mission goal they support.
Within the mission goal of delivering healthcare value, the measures are
further subdivided by domain of value. Each individual measure is equally
weighted to maintain maximum network flexibility and to encourage strategic
network system thinking.

INSTRUCTIONS FOR A: The Core Competencies are designed to evaluate
the executive. What actions has the Network Director taken *personally* to effect
positive change and improve overall Network performance in each area of
competency? Each section has 'bullets' that, as appropriate, should be
addressed in the body of the evaluation of that section and must be sufficiently
descriptive to assess executive performance. (I.e. This self-evaluation is not
intended to be a description of the Network's accomplishments in general but
rather the individual and specific actions and behaviors of the Network
Director that contributed to those accomplishments.) The actions displayed
are not intended to be exclusive. Network Directors should feel free to add
alternative 'bullets' that support specific Network initiatives. In addition,
during the negotiation of this Performance Plan, any individual areas of

emphasis, that past performance may indicate are necessary will be added to the "core" set of competencies listed.

Part A   Core Competencies[1]

VHA Strategic Enabling Goal: Deliver world-class service to veterans and their families by applying sound business principles that result in effective management of people, communications, technology, and governance
Objective: Improve the overall governance and performance of VA by applying sound business principles and ensuring accountability
Baldrige: Leadership

Part A – Section 1: 30 Percent of Performance Contract

I. **Interpersonal Effectiveness**: The ability to build and sustain relationships, resolves conflicts, handle negotiations effectively, and develop collaborative working relationships. The successful executive displays empathy, empowers others, and possesses written and oral communication skills.

- Through effective communications, builds and maintains effective partnerships and mutually supportive relations with Veteran Service Organizations.
- Provides fair, principled, decisive leadership to facility employees inspiring a climate of productivity, effectiveness and high morale.
- Provides for an environment that recognizes all employees as leaders and promotes the concepts of shared leadership and accountability.
- Maintains effective relations with the public and media, which results in a positive image of VA in the network or the community.
- Promotes an effective, balanced relationship with academic affiliates that results in joint and mutually advantageous partnership. Articulates facility needs; evaluates program; and resolves problem areas.

II. **Systems Thinking**: The ability to understand the pieces as a whole and appreciate the consequences of actions on other parts of the system. The successful executive thinks in context, knows how to link actions with others in the organization and demonstrates awareness of process, procedures and outcomes. (S/he) possesses a big (whole) picture view of the world.

- Develops and implements network business plan on timely basis.
- Effectively supports VHA and Network initiatives; identifies unique opportunities to expand quality, access, and timeliness of care to veterans.

---

1 Critical Success Factor

Syracuse VA continued

- Identifies opportunities to strengthen Network through local programs; communicates and defends initiatives to consolidate or integrate services and facilities.
- Develops effective sharing and partnership agreements with local institutions.

III. **Flexibility/Adaptability**: The ability to quickly adapt to change, handle multiple inputs and tasks simultaneously and accommodate new situations and realities. The successful executive works well with all levels and types of people, welcomes divergent ideas and maximizes limited resources.

- Allocates resources, including funds, staff, equipment and plant, in an effective manner responding to changes in budget plan, construction issues, VHA and Network priorities, etc. Utilizes full range of approaches including contracts, sharing agreements, etc. to achieve desired outcomes.
- Balances various stakeholder needs, including those of patients, staff, affiliates, Labor Partnership and Veterans Service Organizations to optimize outcomes.

IV. **Organizational Stewardship**: The successful executive is sensitive to the needs of individuals and the organization and provides service to both. (S/he) assumes accountability for self, others, and the organization. This executive demonstrates commitment to people and empowers and trusts others.

- Ensures that internal control systems are in place to ensure accountability for funds, equipment, motor vehicles, and other assets.
- Operates an effective Compliance Program.
- Balances organization's needs and resources to effectively carry out the multiple missions of the organization.
- *Ensures that objective requirements of Public Law 107–135 to maintain capacity to provide for the specialized treatment and rehabilitative needs of disabled veterans (including spinal cord dysfunction, blindness, amputations, and mental illness) are met.*[2]
- Communicates network goals, objectives, & achievements to internal & external stakeholders.
- Implements effective affirmative action program within network.
- Ensures diversity in executive level committees at both the network and facility level.
- Takes positive action to identify and resolve grievances/complaints of discrimination.

---

2 New to Part A in FY03.

Syracuse VA continued

- Implements a system to communicate organization expectations and standards of conduct. Holds supervisors & employees accountable for performance and behavior.

- Operates an effective safety & occupational health program that meets VA, JCAHO, and OSHA standards.

- *Operates an effective healthcare environmental program to provide and maintain a clean, safe and sanitary environment that is in compliance with VA, JCAHO, EPA, and industry best practices.*[3]

- Exercises due diligence or care in efforts to plan, develop, coordinate, and implement an effective information security program.

Part A Section 2[4]: 20 Percent of Performance Contract

I. **Service**: The ability to integrate service to veterans and others, including patient satisfaction and stakeholder support, into a management plan. A service-driven executive enhances internal and external satisfaction. (S/he) models service by handling complaints effectively and promptly and ensuring a patient-centered focus in direction and daily work. This executive uses patient and other stakeholder feedback in planning and providing products and services and encourages subordinates to meet or exceed patient and stakeholder needs and expectations.

- Operates an effective program to receive, evaluate and resolve patient-initiated complaints. Tracks data to identify and correct systemic issues.

- Fosters a patient-focused environment resulting in demonstrable improvements in patient service outcomes.

II. **Creative Thinking**: The ability to think and act innovatively, look beyond current reality to forecast future direction, take risks, challenge traditional assumptions and solve problems creatively. The successful executive is resourceful.

- Identifies, develops, and implements alternative organizational structures to accomplish mission.

- Identifies innovative ways to make optimal use of limited resources in establishing high priority programs.

- Identifies opportunities to partner with other organizations to improve service.

---

3 New Performance Plan in FY03
4 Critical Success Factor

III. **Personal Mastery**: The ability to recognize personal strengths and weaknesses and to engage in continuous learning and self-development. The successful executive demonstrates a willingness to take actions to change, and takes charge of own career.

- Participates in significant professional activities including appropriate certification.

IV. **Technical**: The knowledge and skills to perform and evaluate the work of the organization based upon a clear understanding of the processes, procedures, standards, methods, and technologies of the organization. The successful executive demonstrates functional and technical literacy and measures results of work.

- Ensures the implementation of effective programs to ensure high quality care.
- Ensures appropriate medical record documentation monitoring mechanisms are maintained for record review and problem identification and resolution.
- Ensures that the elements of the High Performance Development Program are fully implemented.
- Ensures the full impact of construction projects on existing facilities is considered and planned for, as: interruption of patient care services, utility shutdowns, impact on employee working conditions, etc. Ensures appropriate measures are taken to mitigate any adverse impacts.
- Establishes and ensures substantial achievement of contracting goals for small business (8a), minority and women contractors for his/her network. Provides necessary resources and personal support to ensure that Acquisition staff is provided maximum opportunity to achieve the established Department goals for purchases from small, minority, women and veteran owned business.

PART B: Performance Measures (50 Percent of Performance Contract)

HEALTHCARE VALUE: Domain of Quality

VHA Strategic Goal 3: Honor and serve veterans in life and memorialize them in death for their sacrifices on behalf of the Nation
Objective: Provide high quality, reliable, accessible, timely and efficient health care that maximizes the health and functional status for all enrolled veterans, with priority access to veterans with service-connected conditions, those unable to defray the cost, and those statutorily eligible for care.
Baldrige 7.1: Organizational Performance Results – Patient Focused Results

Clinical Interventions:

By the end of FY03, Network Directors and Program Officials will assure that the percent of patients in compliance with appropriate clinical interventions will increase. There are seven measures in this section; each will be displayed in a quadrant format demonstrating improvement over time and performance compared to individual targets.

Measure 1: Cancer

A. Percent of patients receiving:
   i) Screening for Breast Cancer
   ii) Screening for Cervical Cancer
   iii) Screening for Colorectal Cancer
   iv) Education for Prostate Cancer Screening

Measure 2: Cardiovascular

1. Heart Failure – Ambulatory Care: Percent of patients admitted for HF and:
   a. On ACEI prior to admission
   b. On beta blocker prior to admission
   c. Receiving weight monitoring instruction prior to admission
2. Heart Failure – Inpatients: Percent of inpatients with primary HF diagnosis and:
   a. LVEF assessment prior to discharge
   b. LVEF <40 on an ACE inhibitor (JCAHO Core)
   c. On a beta-blocker agent
   d. Receiving discharge instructions that include information regarding diet, weight, medications and follow up care (JCAHO Core)
3. Hypertension: Percent of patients with diagnosis of hypertension and:
   a. BP less than or equal to 140/90
   b. BP greater than or equal to 160/90
4. Ischemic Heart Disease–Ambulatory: Percent of patients with AMI in past 5 yrs AND:
   a. LDL-c <120 mg/dL (Most recent test in past 2 years)
   b. ASA on last visit
   c. Beta Blocker on last visit
5. Ischemic Heart Disease–Inpatient: Percent of Acute Myocardial Infarction Inpatients and:
   a. B-blocker @ arrival (JCAHO Core)
   b. Applicable AMI patients who receive reperfusion (baseline to be 1st qtr, performance period to be Qtrs 2,3 & 4)
   c. Diagnosis LV dysfunction whose qualitative EF assessment is completed prior to discharge.
   d. With LVEF<40 that are receiving Ace inhibitors (JCAHO Core)

Measure 3: Endocrinology

1. Percent of patients with Diabetes Mellitus and:
   a. Eye examination at the appropriate interval
   b. Glycemic control – HBA1c <9
   c. Glycemic control – HBA1c >11 or not done (lower number is better)
   d. HTN BP less than or equal to 140/90

    e. HTN BP >160/90 (lower number is better)

    f. LDL-C <120 mg/dL. (Most recent test in past 2 years)

Measure 4: Infectious

1. Hepatitis C: Percent of patients in each of two cohorts; a. Primary Care and b. Mental Health Diagnosis:

    a. Screened

    b. Tested

    c. With positive risk factors but not tested (lower number is better)

2. Immunizations: Percent of applicable patients in each of two cohorts; a. Primary Care and b. Spinal Cord Injury & Disorders receiving immunizations for:

    a. Influenza

    b. Pneumococcal

Measure 5: Mental Health

1. Major Depressive Disorder: Percent of patients:

    a. Screened for depression

    b. With positive screen that receive follow-up within six weeks.

2. Substance Use Disorder: Percent of patients:

    a. Screened for problem alcohol usage

    b. Beginning a new episode of designated substance abuse treatment who maintain continuous treatment involvement for at least 90 days

Measure 6: Tobacco: Percent of patients:

1. In three patient cohorts; a. Primary Care, b. Mental Health Diagnosis, and c. Spinal Cord Injury & Disorders:

    a. Screened for Tobacco Use

2. Of those using tobacco, percent of patients:

    a. Counseled at least 3 times in the past 12 months to stop

    b. Having used tobacco in the past 12 months. (Compatible with Health People 2010, CDC NCHS, and JCAHO) Lower number is better; segmented by a) cigarettes or b) other tobacco products

3. With inpatient discharge for Heart Failure receiving Tobacco cessation counseling while inpatient (JCAHO Core)

4. With inpatient discharge for Acute Myocardial Infarction receiving Tobacco cessation counseling while inpatient (JCAHO Core)

5. With inpatient discharge for Community Acquired Pneumonia receiving Tobacco cessation counseling while inpatient (JCAHO Core)

Measure 7: Respiratory

Percent of patients with an inpatient episode of care for Bacterial pneumonia and:

    1) Pneumococcal immunization any time prior to admission

    2) Influenza immunization - during the previous flu season (and prior to admission)

3) O2 assessment with ABG or pulse oximetry within 24 hrs of arrival (JCAHO Core)
4) Blood cultures collected before first antibiotic dose (JCAHO Core)

VA Strategic Objective: Implement a One VA information technology framework that supports the integration of information across business lines and that provides a source of consistent, reliable, accurate, and secure information to veterans and their families, employees, and stakeholders

Measure 8: Patient Safety

By end of FY03, percent of patches to CPRS, Imaging and BCMA software installed within appropriate time period will increase.

Measure 9: CPRS

By 4th Qtr FY03, Provider Order Entry of New Pharmacy Orders will maintain or achieve target.

HEALTHCARE VALUE: FUNCTION

VA Strategic Goal 1: Restore the capability of veterans with disabilities to the greatest extent possible and improve the quality of their lives and that of their families
Strategic Objective: Maximize the physical, mental, and social functioning of veterans with disabilities and be recognized as a leader in the provision of specialized health care services

Measure 10: Rehabilitation

By end of FY03, the percent of patients with new stroke, amputations, or traumatic brain injury with initial Functional Independence Measure (FIM) assessment and entered into FSOD will increase.

Measure 11: Homeless

By end of FY03 the percent of veterans discharged from:
  i. Domiciliary Care for Homeless Veterans (DCHV) Program or
  ii. Health Care for Homeless Veterans (HCHV) Community based contract residential care program, or
  iii. Grant Per Diem Homeless care to independent housing or a secure institutional arrangement will increase.

HEALTHCARE VALUE: SATISFACTION

VHA Strategic Goal 3: Honor and serve veterans in life and memorialize them in death for their sacrifices on behalf of the Nation
Objective: Provide high quality, reliable, accessible, timely and efficient health care that maximizes the health and functional status for all enrolled veterans, with priority access to veterans with service-connected conditions, those unable to defray the cost, and those statutorily eligible for care.

Measure 12: Patient Satisfaction:
By end of FY03 the percent of patients reporting overall satisfaction as Very Good or Excellent will increase in:
a. Ambulatory Care: For patients seen in Quarters 1, 2, & 3
b. Inpatient: For patients discharged in Quarters 1, 2, and 3

Employer of Choice:
VA Strategic Enabling Goal: Deliver work-class service to veterans and their families by applying sound business principles that result in effective management of people, communications, technology, and governance
Strategic Objective: Recruit, develop, and retain a competent, committed, and diverse workforce that provides high quality service to veterans and their families

Measure 13: Employee Satisfaction:
By end of FY03, VISN will have made progress toward achieving milestones developed in FY02 Employee Satisfaction Plan

Measure 14: Work Force Planning:
By the end of FY03, Network Directors and Program Officials will assure that strategic plans for their organization contain a workforce and leadership development plan that meets the following criteria:
1. The strategic plan contains a component addressing workforce development including a succession plan that identifies projected workforce needs and underrepresented employee groups by occupation as well as goals and objectives to guide diversity management, education and HPDM plans.
2. Workforce and leadership development programs are linked to the strategic goals and objectives that:
   a. Provide a process to identify diverse groups of high potential employees,
   b. Provide for an active Diversity Advisory Committee or similar structure in the Network (or at each facility) and Program Office
   c. Offer an organization-wide developmental mentoring program to employees
   d. Maintain formal recruitment relationships such as cooperative education or intern programs with at least two minority-serving institutions, e.g. HBCU or HACU as geographically appropriate,
   e. Provide for a mechanism to regularly analyze employee satisfaction data and addresses causes of significant dissatisfiers
   f. Provide for at least three clearly defined on-going programs offering wide developmental opportunities available to the workforce

HEALTHCARE VALUE: ACCESS

VA Strategic Goal 1: Restore the capability of veterans with disabilities to the greatest extent possible and improve the quality of their lives and that of their families

Syracuse VA continued

Strategic Objective: Maximize the physical, mental, and social functioning of veterans with disabilities and be recognized as a leader in the provisions of specialized health care services

Measure 15: Mental Health:

By end of FY03 the percent high risk patients screened for Mental Health Intensive Case Management (MHICM) will increase.

Wait Times:
VA Strategic Goal 3: Honor and serve veterans in life and memorialize them in death for their sacrifices on behalf of the Nation
Strategic Objective: Provide high quality, reliable, accessible, timely and efficient health care that maximizes the health and functional status for all enrolled veterans, with priority access to veterans with service-connected conditions, those unable to defray the cost, and those statutorily eligible for care

Measure 16: Waiting times – Clinic

By September 30, 2003 Networks will improve waiting time for key clinics as measured by a combination of indicators to include:

a. Primary Care – New Patients: Percent of new patents at 3rd Qtr of the SHEP Survey who answer "yes" to the question, "Did you get an appointment when you wanted one?" Target – 79%
b. Primary Care – Established Patients: Percent of established patents at 3rd Qtr of the SHEP Survey who answer "yes" to the question, "Did you get an appointment when you wanted one?" Target 79%
c. Specialty Care - Wait time from date entered into scheduling package until date of appointment for 'Next Available Appointment', in September 2003 for patients in: (all individual targets must be met)
   i. Eye care – Target 63 days or less
   ii. Urology – Target 44 days or less
   iii. Orthopedics – Target 43 days or less
   iv. Audiology – Target 40 days or less
   v. Cardiology – Target 42 days or less

Measure 17: Waiting times - Provider

By 3rd Qtr, 2003, percent of patients who report in the Survey of Healthcare Experience of Patients (SHEP) Ambulatory Care Survey waiting for a provider 20 minutes or less will increase.

HEALTHCARE VALUE: Cost

VA Strategic Enabling Goal: Deliver work-class service to veterans and their families by applying sound business principles that result in effective management of people, communications, technology, and governance
Strategic Objective: Improve the overall governance and performance of VA by applying sound business principles and ensuring accountability

Measure 18: Revenue

1. By the end of FY03 for 2nd–4th Qtr the percent of dollars in AR < 90 days will increase.
2. By the end of FY03 for 2nd–4th Qtr the timeliness will increase for the following:
   a. Inpatient:
      i. Generation of inpatient claim
      ii. Collection of inpatient claim
   b. Outpatient:
      i. Generating outpatient bill
      ii. Collection of outpatient bill
3. By the end of FY03 for 2nd–4th Qtr the adjusted billed (claim) to collected ratio will increase. *(Pending final review Nov 1, 2002)*

HEALTHCARE VALUE: BUILDING HEALTHY COMMUNITIES:

VA Strategic Goal 4: Contribute to the public health, emergency management, socioeconomic well-being, and history of the Nation
Strategic Objective: Advance VA medical research and development programs that address veterans' needs, with an emphasis on service-connected injuries and illnesses, and contribute to the Nation's knowledge of disease and disability

Measure 19: Research: Accreditation

By September 30, 2003, all Research Programs subject to NCQA survey in FY2003, for Human Research Protection will receive Accreditation or Conditional Accreditation.

FY2003 PERFORMANCE AGREEMENT

_____   _____
Network Director   Date

_____   _____
Laura J. Miller   Date
Deputy Under Secretary for Health
for Operations and Management

_____   _____
Robert H. Roswell, MD   Date
Under Secretary for Health (10)

CASE STUDY 4.3: Chesapeake General Hospital, Chesapeake, VA   (Reprinted with permission)

MEMORANDUM

TO: Members of the Chesapeake Hospital Authority

FROM: Donald S. Buckley, Ph.D., President

DATE: September 27, 2001

SUBJECT: EVALUATION OF PRESIDENT, CEO

The material in this booklet is prepared for the Chesapeake Hospital Authority's use in conducting my annual evaluation.

The following elements of the operation of Chesapeake Health and Chesapeake General Hospital are presented for your review in this process:

Chesapeake Health Family
Financial Review
Medical Staff Relations
Patient Satisfaction
Employee Relations
Quality and Cost Enhancements
Community Outreach
Goals and Objectives Fiscal Year 2001
Accomplishments Not Included in Goals and Objectives
Status Report of Activities and Projects in Fiscal year 2001
Strategic Planning
State of Chesapeake Health

Literature Review on Hospital CEO Performance Evaluation, 1994–2001

Compiled by Ritu Jain

2001

*Flynn, P. 2001. "You Are Simply Average." *Across the Board* (March/April): 51–55.

This article illustrates two functions of performance appraisals—comparative rating and performance/job management. The author argues for the separation of these two functions during the yearly performance appraisal. Comparing an individual's relative strengths and weaknesses to others is a difficult process psychologically for managers and employees. This is especially true because the majority of employees fall in the middle, "you are average" category. The good, but average, performer does not need to be told every year that they are average. Contrary to the comparative rating that takes place once a year, the job management/goal-setting message needs to be relayed more frequently than that. Goals, achievements, and opportunities for performance and job improvement should be discussed without comparison to others.

*Miller, J. S., and F. A. Rosland. 2001. "Person Versus System: Situational Constraints and Appraisal Satisfaction." Paper presented at the 61st Annual Meeting of the Academy of Management, Washington, DC.

This study investigated appraisal satisfaction among 265 employees of six nonprofits and one business organization. It examined the effects of system factors on survey respondents' level of satisfaction with the appraisal process. Worker satisfaction with the appraisal is vital for motivating employees and for long-term effectiveness. Three systems factors are studied: situational constraints, coworker relations, and communication quality. The research shows that appraisal satisfaction is significantly higher when situational constraints

---

* Not specific to healthcare management

are minimized and when positive workplace communication and positive relationships with colleagues are present. Holding individuals accountable for performance when system factors, over which employees have no control, strongly influence outcomes and detracts from fairness perceptions.

*Neal, J. E. 2001. *The #1 Guide to Performance Appraisals. Doing It Right!* Ohio: Neal Publishers, Inc.

This concise book provides tips for effectively developing, completing, and administering performance appraisals. The author suggests that upper management evaluations should be based on factors such as earnings, sales, vision, leadership, strategic planning, organizing, communications, and management succession. He comments that the growing number of employment contracts at high management levels may negate the use of performance appraisals. This guide is principally devoted to developing performance appraisals for mid-level employees and staff.

Newman, J. F., L. Tyler, and D. M. Dunbar. 2001. "CEO Performance Appraisal: Review and Recommendations." *Journal of Healthcare Management* 46 (1): 21–38.

This article discusses several problems with CEO performance appraisals and offers contemporary approaches to improve the process. Three areas of evaluation are organizational success, areawide health status, and professional role fulfillment. The article argues that the final goal of appraisals is to link results to incentive compensation and recommends that some portion of the CEO's salary hinge on performance in two critical areas: organizational effectiveness and community health status. The evaluation process can be initiated by the board or the CEO, by a committee, or by an outside consultant. In highly political situations, the outside consultant is recommended. Some novel ideas introduced in the article include the suggestion that the 360-degree feedback should be provided by a counselor who will develop a personal action plan with the CEO. Three functional areas should form the basis for evaluations: (1) position description; (2) strategic plan; and (3) the organization's mission statement, although this is difficult to measure objectively.

Oliveira, J. 2001. "The Balanced Scorecard: An Integrative Approach to Performance Evaluation." *Healthcare Financial Management* 55 (5): 42–46.

In addition to financial performance, intangible assets that affect a company's bottom line should also be assessed. The balanced scorecard developed by Robert Kaplan and David Norton is a way of addressing this performance-measurement limitation. The approach encourages behavioral changes aimed at achieving corporate strategies. It suggests specific indicators that managers and staff can influence directly by their actions. The four indicators are long-term financial performance, staff development, internal efficiency, and customer satisfaction. The scorecard ties each corporate objective to an outcome measurement. The objectives are associated with a "driver" that enables the achievement of the objective. The cause-and-effect relationship of the outcome and driver measurements allows managers to develop actions aimed at improving performance. Outlined in the article are ten steps to create the balanced scorecard framework and the kinds of information needed for such an analysis.

*Peiperl, M. A. 2001. "Best Practice. Getting 360-degree Feedback Right." *Harvard Business Review* (January): 142–47.

This article discusses research conducted on the theory and practice of 360-degree feedback. The author studied 17 companies varying in size and industry and found four inescapable paradoxes embedded in the process:
1. Paradoxes of roles: employees are torn between being supportive of colleagues and judging them.
2. Paradox of group performance: appraising individuals ignores group dynamics and group work and threatens group performance.
3. Measurement paradox: numerical ratings do not allow for qualitative comments and insights, which are difficult and time consuming.
4. Paradoxes of rewards: employees become more keenly attuned to peer appraisals when they affect salary and promotions. Attention is focused on rewards rather than on constructive feedback.

Tyler, L. J., and E. Biggs. 2001. "Practical Governance: CEO Performance Appraisal." *Trustee* 54 (5): 18–21.

This article offers suggestions to trustees on how to make CEO appraisals more fair and beneficial. Some factors that hinder a board from facilitating a good performance appraisal include fear of confrontation, lack of clarity over priorities, failure to specify a job description, uncertainty regarding the appropriate criteria to be used in assessment, and overall concern that the special CEO-board relationship will be disturbed. The objective of the performance appraisal process is to support or change behavior. Some ways that boards can increase the effectiveness of appraisals are using a 360-degree feedback rater system and providing regular feedback. Both the CEO's job description and the hospital's mission should be reviewed during the appraisal. The article also lists determinants of CEO compensation such as an organization's performance, benchmarking salary, equity within the organization, inflation, length of time in position, risk or volatility of position, and political or community considerations.

Weber, D. O. 2001. "A Better Gauge of Corporate Performance." *Health Forum Journal* 44 (3): 20–24.

This article describes how the Kaplan-Norton balanced scorecard concept came about. The model functions on four key perspectives—financial strength, customer service and satisfaction, internal operating efficiency, and learning and growth. Under each perspective are key measures constituting a unified strategic goal. Healthcare organizations are distinguished from other types of organizations because of the complexity of their mission and their constituents and the nature of their product. Healthcare settings have focused heavily on nonfinancial measurements of performance. Because putting a value on human life is difficult, the scorecard concept has been slow in being adopted.

Alexander, J. A., B. J. Weiner, and M. Succi. 2000. "Community Accountability Among Hospitals Affiliated with Health Care Systems." *The Milbank Quarterly* 78 (2): 149, 157–84.

This article examines how community accountability differs between system-affiliated hospitals and freestanding hospitals and whether community accountability differs in degree or form across hospitals affiliated with different types of systems. Based on results from the American Hospital Association's 1997 Hospital Governance Survey (a national survey of 2,079 hospitals with a 42 percent response rate), comparisons are made in how hospitals in each category exercise community accountability in the composition, structure, and activity of their governing boards. Hospitals' exercise of community accountability is classified into three categories: (1) the presence and structure of a community-based hospital board, (2) the existence of initiatives for monitoring and reporting information about community health and hospital performance, and (3) collaboration with other local agencies to enhance community benefits. Boards of system-affiliated hospitals are more likely than freestanding hospital boards to perform certain types of evaluation on a routine basis—that is, evaluate the CEO on community health improvements. Boards of system-affiliated hospitals exercise community accountability most strongly in their information monitoring and reporting activities, whereas freestanding hospitals exercise community accountability through the structural and compositional attributes of their boards.

*Crane, J. S., and N. K. Crane. 2000. "A Multi-Level Performance Appraisal Tool: Transition from the Traditional to a CQI Approach." *Health Care Management Review* 25 (1): 64–73.

In this case study, a multilevel appraisal model is proposed that enables managers to evaluate organizational progress as a sum of contributions made by each employee's work, performance of quality groups, and achievement of the organizational mission. The model emphasizes the importance of adequate evaluation of group performance as opposed to the traditional appraisal of individual performance. The model was tested in a pharmaceutical company committed to continuous quality improvement. To objectively assess the internal and external performance of an organization, placing emphasis on the system and its processes, not the individual, is essential. A true quality appraisal system emphasizes intrinsic motivators and views employees as capable, self-actualizing individuals. This research shows that pay for performance frequently fails as a motivator because it is unable to measure and document performance differentials accurately and completely.

*DeNisi, A. S., and A. N. Kluger. 2000. "Feedback Effectiveness: Can 360-degree Appraisals Be Improved?" *Academy of Management Executive* 14 (1): 129–39.

This review article cites empirical research showing that although nearly two-thirds of feedback improves performance, more than one-third of feedback actually lowers subsequent performance. The specific conditions under which feedback might be more effective are discussed. For example, feedback should be given at the end of a complex task not in the middle of it, providing feedback about past performance that has improved over time tends to increase subsequent performance, and computer-generated feedback increases the effectiveness of feedback. Including specific recommendations for improvement is more likely to be effective in improving performance, and goal setting should accompany feedback. The authors suggest that feedback should focus on the task and task performance only, not on the person or any part of the person's self-concept. Feedback should minimize information concerning the relative performance of others.

The authors then consider the 360-degree feedback specifically. Designed to ask raters to provide evaluations in areas where they are qualified to make judgments, this type of feedback was originally instituted for developmental purposes. Aspects of the system that make this type of feedback less effective are using them only once, focusing on the self instead of tasks, not including goal setting, and not providing information about correct solutions. The 360-degree appraisal should not be used for decision making, be certain to interpret the results and permit reactions, and avoid having all raters evaluate employees in all areas. Consider a personal coach to help interpret results, include goal setting, and use the 360-degree feedback regularly.

*Ghorpade, J. 2000. "Managing Five Paradoxes of 360-degree Feedback." *Academy of Management Executive* 14 (1): 140–50.

A 360-degree feedback program enables organizational members to receive feedback on their performance from all major constituencies they serve. The authors of the article argue that the 360-degree method is filled with paradoxes and has serious problems relating to privacy, validity, and effectiveness. Five paradoxes exist around four issues involved in the adoption of the feedback system: objectives, sources of behavior and performance data, methods of data gathering and feedback, and selection of a program administrator. These paradoxes are as follows:

1. Employee development paradox: 360-degree feedback is used as an appraisal tool rather than a developmental one.
2. Multiple constituents paradox: increasing the number of raters does not increase the quality of the feedback.
3. Anonymous ratings paradox: honest ratings are not necessarily the most valid. Biases—including halo effect, self-serving bias, and leniency—can distort accuracy.
4. Structured feedback paradox: a 360-degree feedback tool should balance quantitative rating with qualitative data. Behaviors involved in a job are difficult to measure.
5. Managerial involvement paradox: managerial involvement in gathering and processing the feedback may taint the process. Feedback receivers should trust the feedback's administrator.

The article offers solutions on how to manage these five problems when using the 360-degree feedback tool.

Hawthorne, G. W., and C. J. Bolster. 2000. "The 10th Annual Compensation and Salary Guide." *Hospitals & Health Networks* 74 (9): 38–46.

HayGroup's Compensation Survey shows that the base median CEO salary was $216,600 in 2000, compared to $180,000 in 1999. The total median compensation is $230,000 per year. Bonuses make up an average of 32 percent of the CEOS' base salaries. Of the surveyed organizations, 65 percent report the use of performance-based incentive programs, up by 59 percent from 1999. Only 10 percent report the use of long-term incentives, which are typically used as a retention vehicle.

*Scullen, S. E., M. K. Mount, and M. Goff. 2000. "Understanding the Latent Structure of Job Performance Ratings." *Journal of Applied Psychology* 85 (6): 956–70.

This study examined 2,350 managers, and another separate analysis of 2,142 managers, from various industries and at different levels in their organizations' hierarchy. They were subjected to a 360-degree feedback process by two bosses, two peers, two subordinates, and self. The study found that the ratings received were mostly the result of idiosyncratic rater effects instead of general and specific dimensional performance. Of the various raters, bosses' ratings captured more of the actual job performance measures than those of peers or subordinates. Performance ratings are used in practice to make decisions concerning pay raises, promotions, and terminations. Results show that a greater proportion of variance in ratings is associated with biases of the rater rather than with the performance of the ratee.

1999

Bogue, R. J. 1999. "An Incentive for Community Health. Linking CEO Compensation to Community Goals." *Trustee* 52 (5): 15–19.

Targeted at trustees, this article lists ten reasons for making community health improvement a core business strategy. Some of the reasons are that it reduces costs through health education and prevention and by linking more effectively other health resources in the community and reducing underutilized, duplicate capacity. The article then highlights comments of three hospital CEOs of health systems where compensation tied to community health performance has been successfully implemented.

Devan, V. R., and M. Williams. 1999. "Measuring Up. Benchmarking Tools Can Enhance Executive Performance." *Trustee* 52 (5): 6–9.

This is an article directed to board members and examines the use of benchmarking as a tool to evaluate executive performance. Healthcare organizations should use external sources to find data, and trustees must recognize the different types of benchmarking data. Trustees and the CEO must agree on specific, measurable goals defined by benchmarking data. Financial indicators that can be benchmarked are labor cost per adjusted discharge, nonlabor cost per adjusted discharge, revenue measurements, professional fees, capital cost per adjusted discharge, and clinical utilization cost per adjusted discharge. Boards can track the overall performance of the organization this way.

Milstead, L. 1999. "The Pressure Is On: Tying Executive Pay to Community Benefits." *Health Forum Journal* 42 (2): 47–49.

Tax-exempt hospitals and health systems are missing an important opportunity to align executive compensation with the need of their community. The author describes a 1998 Court of Appeals decision in Pennsylvania where the court upheld the revocation of Harrisburg Hospital's property tax exemption because some of the hospital's operations were found to indicate a private profit motive. This case sends a clear message, claims the author, that compensation for executives needs to be tied to community-benefit objectives. Because not-for-profit hospitals provide care for the underinsured and uninsured, they are typically exempt from federal, state, and local taxes. But these laws require reporting of the community benefits they provide and justification for exemption. The author makes the point that some hospitals do not have reliable systems to measure benefits, which are critical for tying executive pay to this area of performance. Currently, most hospitals can measure community benefits only as activities performed and are unable to measure the results or outcomes of these activities.

Wolper, L. F. 1999. *Health Care Administration*, 3rd edition. New York: Aspen Publishers.

Trustees have an obligation to hire and then evaluate the competency of CEOs. Appraisal systems evaluate an employee's work by comparing actual with expected performance. Appraisals have many uses, including the following:
1. Determining whether the CEO's work results are consistent with expectations
2. Providing feedback to the CEO as well as the board
3. Identifying acceptable and unsatisfactory behaviors
4. Assessing CEO performance levels (less-than-satisfactory performance may be a result of employee variables such as skills or experience, systems processes, or job design)
5. Providing information for compensation
6. Providing information for employee assistance

Therefore, control over performance appraisals and information-gathering systems are of great importance.

1998

*Kirkland, K., and S. Manoogian. 1998. *Ongoing Feedback. How to Get It, How to Use It*. Ideas Into Action Guidebook. Greensboro, NC: Center for Creative Leadership.

Suggestions are provided on how to choose a peer reviewer for the 360-feedback assessment; a reviewer should have an interest in your effectiveness and should be able to speak to you directly and honestly. Suggestions are also given as to when you should ask for a review; an assessment is due after you have identified your goals. Set a time limit for achieving your goals. Ask for feedback daily from your peers and coworkers so you can put your goals into action. The crux of this guidebook is how to ask for feedback. The Situation-Behavior-Impact (SBI) model gives reviewers a framework for structuring their information and perceptions of you, and it provides a safe way for others to give feedback. The model breaks down the perception of your performance into three areas: (1) describing the situation, (2) describing your behavior, and (3) describing the impact that your behavior had on other people. The authors also offer some dos and don'ts when using the SBI model. Example of dos are explain how you would like to receive your feedback, listen, and pay attention to nonverbal responses. An example of don't is not to become defensive or to judge the value of the feedback when it is being given.

Manion, J. 1998. *From Management to Leadership. Interpersonal Skills for Success in Health Care.* Chicago: American Hospital Publishers, Inc.

The author identifies the fundamental interpersonal competencies every leader needs such as trust, mutual respect, and communication. Suggestions are offered for improving these skills. The author explores the difference between management and leadership, the relationship between leader and follower, how to build commitment among followers, clear communication, how to develop others, and the principles of the managing process.

Olden, P. C., and D. G. Clement. 1998. "Well-Being Revisited: Improving the Health of a Population." *Journal of Healthcare Management* 43 (1): 36–50.

This article addresses three issues. First, it differentiates between the words "health" and "medical care." Second, it attempts to clarify what determines the health of a population. Third, it offers advice to healthcare executives and their organizations to improve and maintain the health of a population. Pioneering work that is meant to improve their local environment is presented by several hospitals. Managers should (1) embrace "health" rather than just "medical services," (2) collaborate with other organizations and people to build partnerships, (3) provide some resources and funds to improve health and should view this commitment as an investment, (4) obtain public and private grant funds, and (5) advocate and support public policy.

Proenca, E. J. 1998. "Community Orientation in Health Services Organizations: The Concept and Its Implementation." *Health Care Management Review* 23 (2): 28–38.

This article, drawing from literature in healthcare, presents the concept of community orientation that healthcare organizations can use to provide community-focused care. Community orientation is described as the performance of three activities: (1) the generation of intelligence on current and future community health needs, (2) the dissemination of such intelligence across the organization and into the community, and (3) coordination of an interdepartmental and interinstitutional response to it. Orientation can be achieved when front-line employees and community representative are involved in environmental analysis, when evaluation and reward systems are based on community health outcomes, and when internal information systems are integrated into community health information networks. Greater market share, better cost and quality outcomes, superior performance, and satisfied stakeholders are given as reasons for hospitals to develop a high degree of community orientation.

*Tornow, W. W., and M. London. 1998. *Maximizing the Value of 360-Degree Feedback*. Greensboro, NC: Center for Creative Leadership and Jossey-Bass.

Written by several authors, all of whom were associated with the Center for Creative Leadership, this article presents a common theme: 360-degree feedback can promote individual development and improve individual performance if the feedback is linked to developmental planning, goal setting, and organizational support. Four conditions will maximize the value of the 360-degree feedback process: (1) the intervention is business driven, (2) the organization needs the measured behaviors, (3) the survey instrument is reliable and valid, (4) and the conditions for learning new skills exist.

1997

Hofrichter, D. A., and G. W. Hawthorne. 1997. "Governing Performance. Reexamining the Board's Role in Executive Compensation." *Trustee* 50 (6): 7–12.

This article focuses the board's attention on the growing importance of executive and physician incentive pay and compensation. The 1996 Total Compensation Survey by the HayGroup showed that annual incentive plans are common among healthcare systems. This article outlines five steps trustees can take to be more active in setting executive compensation packages. First, create an independent compensation committee. Second, develop a sound compensation philosophy that is in line with the organization's culture, mission, and business strategy. Third, develop a sound policy to support that philosophy. Fourth, review your executive compensation program on a regular basis. Fifth, use reliable compensation information.

Speer, T. L. 1997. "Paid to Produce. More and More CEOs Are Accountable for Community Health with Their Paychecks." *Hospitals & Health Networks* 71 (10): 50, 52, 54.

This article looks at four health systems: Crozer-Keystone Health System (Philadelphia), MCG Healthcare (Minneapolis), Lutheran Health System (North Dakota), and the Cambridge Public Health commission. These four are pioneers in linking community health with executive compensation. Measurements are taken in the areas of violence prevention, immunizations, prenatal care, substance abuse, smoking cessation and prevention programs, number of mammograms, and HIV and sexually transmitted diseases. The move toward capitated payments makes serving a healthier community a better business proposition. Organizational influence in affecting areawide health status is minimal because the healthcare system accounts for only 10 percent of factors affecting community health.

1996

Orlikoff, J. E., and M. K. Totten. 1996. "CEO Evaluation and Compensation" Workbook. *Trustee* 49 (1): suppl 4p.

This workbook article outlines for a hospital board the purposes and benefits of the CEO evaluation process. It details three elements of the evaluation process. First, evaluations should flow from a written compensation philosophy. Second, boards should have a formal compensation committee that evaluates CEO and other executives. Third, the committee should report to the full board at least annually. The article also outlines certain paradigm shifts occurring in healthcare and how this shift dictates changes in the CEO evaluation process, such as the need for employment contracts and tying compensation to community health.

1994

Pryor, K. T. 1994. "Letter to the Chairman of the Board: Reflections on CEO Evaluations." *Trustee* 47 (4): 22–23.

The former president and CEO of Berkshire Health Systems, the author of this article, writes a letter to his board recommending changes in the evaluation process. Clarity of goals is important. Four or five major priorities should be well defined and phrased so that they are as objective as possible. The board and the CEO must have a clear understanding of what is subjective and what is not. Annual profit-and-loss figures should be replaced with return on investment figures as a better indicator of financial success. The CEO must meet with the board to discuss what type of feedback assessment would be most helpful to both. The author feels that the evaluation process should not be a committee function; the entire board, including community leaders, should be involved. Little evidence supports the idea that pay for performance really increases performance. But if such a program exists, then the board should make the compensation philosophy available to other employees. CEO incentives should not be hidden from community leaders, medical staff, or other employees.

About the Principal Author

Peter A. Weil, Ph.D., FACHE, is vice president of the division of research and development of the American College of Healthcare Executives (ACHE). He conducts periodic surveys to compare executives' careers by gender and race/ethnicity. He also conducts market research to assess members' interest and satisfaction with ACHE's programs and services. Prior to joining ACHE in 1982, Dr. Weil was the director of the National Study of Internal Medicine Manpower based at the University of Chicago; he also taught social epidemiology in the graduate program in hospital and health administration at the University of Chicago. Dr. Weil earned a master's degree in health administration from the University of Iowa and a doctorate in medical sociology from the University of Chicago.